Pediatric Hand Deformities in Occupational Therapy and Physical Therapy

Maren Schelly · Anna-Lena Dunse

Pediatric Hand Deformities in Occupational Therapy and Physical Therapy

Manual Treatment and Splint Therapy

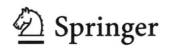
Springer

Maren Schelly
Handchirurgische Abteilung
Katholisches Kinderkrankenhaus
Wilhelmstift
Hamburg, Germany

Anna-Lena Dunse
Handchirurgische Abteilung
Katholisches Kinderkrankenhaus
Wilhelmstift
Hamburg, Germany

Foreword by
Wiebke Hülsemann
Handchirurgische Abteilung
Katholisches Kinderkrankenhaus
Wilhelmstift
Hamburg, Germany

ISBN 978-3-662-68714-7   ISBN 978-3-662-68715-4   (eBook)
https://doi.org/10.1007/978-3-662-68715-4

Translation from the German language edition: "Kindliche Handfehlbildungen in Ergotherapie und Physiotherapie" by Stefanie Gottstein et al., © Der/die Herausgeber bzw. der/die Autor(en), exklusiv lizenziert an Springer-Verlag GmbH, DE, ein Teil von Springer Nature 2023. Published by Springer Berlin Heidelberg. All Rights Reserved.

This book is a translation of the original German edition "Kindliche Handfehlbildungen in Ergotherapie und Physiotherapie" by Stefanie Gottstein, published by Springer-Verlag GmbH, DE in 2023. The translation was done with the help of an artificial intelligence machine translation tool. A subsequent human revision was done primarily in terms of content, so that the book will read stylistically differently from a conventional translation. Springer Nature works continuously to further the development of tools for the production of books and on the related technologies to support the authors.

This Springer imprint is published by the registered company Springer-Verlag GmbH, DE, part of Springer Nature.
The registered company address is: Heidelberger Platz 3, 14197 Berlin, Germany

Paper in this product is recyclable.

Foreword

How would we manage our lives, how would we communicate without our hands? Their perfectly coordinated interplay is a matter of course for us. The hands overcome difficulties so masterfully that we do not think about their abilities. But how do people with malformed hands cope with their everyday life?

Malformations of the upper extremities are rare and vary in complexity. The anatomical changes vary depending on the malformation and the age of the child. The demands children place on their hands depend on the child's age and development. Therefore, treatments must be individually adapted to the malformation, the age, and the development of the child.

The skin of infants and children is thinner, finer, and more elastic than that of adolescents and adults, and it can and must stretch as they grow. The soft tissues have a higher fat content, the bones are soft and consist partly of cartilage depending on the age. In addition, muscular and bony structures can be atrophied, hypertrophied, or otherwise altered due to malformations. After surgical therapy, scar contractures can occur much faster than in adults.

All these circumstances must be considered in both operative and conservative treatment. Therefore, doctors and therapists are called upon to develop individual solutions for the treatment of hand malformations and improvement of hand function, so that the affected children can cope better now and in later life.

The hand surgery department at the Catholic Children's Hospital Wilhelmstift has been specializing in the treatment of hand malformations for decades. In an effort to optimize the treatment of children, individual splints and aids for children with hand malformations of different age groups and sizes have been and continue to be produced and continuously optimized. The fruitful collaboration between us hand surgeons, our pediatric nurse, occupational therapist, and the orthopedic technicians working with us made this possible. For example, preoperatively, better conditions could be achieved for wrist adjustment through radialization in the case of radial longitudinal reduction defect. Postoperative results improved through targeted splints, compression care, and guidance for manual therapy. By starting conservative therapy early (in infancy or toddler age), surgeries could be avoided and hand function could be restored or improved. Patience, empathy, experience, manual skill, and efficient work are required in the treatment of the little patients. Intensive guidance of the parents is also important.

Later in adolescence, the treatment of contractures requires considerably more time and is less successful. Then, the challenge is to motivate the adolescents and integrate the therapy as seamlessly as possible into their everyday life.

We, as a team, would like to pass on the developed techniques and treatment concepts for infants, toddlers, school children, and adolescents with hand deformities. The manual is a "work in progress", a suggestion on how the hand function of the little ones can be improved. These suggestions are not set in stone. We gladly receive feedback, suggestions, and proposals for improvement. Write to us!

Such close cooperation between occupational therapists, pediatric nurses, orthopedic technicians, and doctors is unusual and some things are not provided for in the health insurance billing system. But we do not want to be deterred by this, but rather achieve the best for our little patients. They have a right to it.

We do not want to leave unmentioned the support from our sponsor "Hamburg macht Kinder gesund", to whom we would like to express our heartfelt thanks here!

Chief physician of pediatric   Dr. Wiebke Hülsemann
hand surgery at the Wilhelmstift
Children's Hospital
Hamburg,

Preface

In this book, we describe congenital hand deformities, the recommended conservative therapies, as well as the treatment before and after surgeries.

The contents of this book are to be understood as suggestions and are based on our years of work, experience, and further development.

We gladly accept criticism and suggestions in order to further improve our therapies.

We wish you much success in working with your little patients.

Maren Schelly
Anna-Lena Dunse

Acknowledgment

How do I start with my acknowledgment?

First of all, you came to my mind, you little, very young patients. You have definitely shaped me the most as a pediatric nurse. With your serenity and your self-conception, to accept situations as given and to make the best of them. With your anger, strength, and immense volume, whenever you had to make yourselves heard in a situation that was not so funny for you. From you, I learned serenity and speed at the same time. I had to develop my voice so that your parents could understand me despite your objections. And I learned to "read" you when you were not feeling so well. Many of you have literally grown over my head in the meantime and I am glad about our connection despite the change of perspective. Some of you are currently in the phase of life where the world suddenly turns upside down and everyone around you (especially the adults) has become difficult. I am most impressed by you and your help. You agreed when I needed photos of you to explain developmental and treatment steps to parents who are at the beginning of the treatment and still have to process the pain that their child was born with a malformation, and whose concern for their child dominates a large part of everyday life. Thank you!!

My thanks go to you, Anna-Lena. I have longed for support for our patients and for the expertise of an occupational therapist/hand therapist. Not only do our joint treatments often work without words, but the fact that we have grown together so closely and are a support to each other every second is simply a gift. That we have additionally created this book together is not just the icing on the cake, it is simply fantastic.

Through you, Nicole, we were able to develop the conservative treatments so individually and extensively. I could come to you with any treatment and care idea, it always fell on fertile ground. Thank you for your knowledge, your accuracy, your critical eye, your competence, your reliability, your support, and above all your friendship.

Jonas and Mira, our youngest in the group. You build fantastic hand orthoses and don't let go until perfection is achieved for the little and big patients. We have improved a lot with you in the team, developed new things and thus enabled more effective care for our patients. Thank you for your patience and care towards the little rascals, your thirst for knowledge, your reliability, and your team spirit.

Wiebke, boss, thank you for your trust in my abilities, for the time in which I was and am allowed to learn from you, the exchange of thoughts and discourse. That you challenged and promoted me, listened to my ideas and discussed them with me. For your innovativeness and for paving the way for me as a pediatric nurse specialist.

Mrs. Dür and Mrs. Kania, our editors, thank you for the wonderful phone calls, for the patience and calmness with which you answered all my questions. Nothing better could have happened to me.

In addition, I would like to thank "Hamburg Makes Children Healthy" for their interest and generous financial support.

Beatriz, my special thanks go to you. You made my start in hand surgery easier by sharing your immense knowledge. I could always ask you for help, ask professional questions, and admire your brain, which never got tired of remembering the many patients in a matter of seconds. Despite your well-deserved retirement, you have put this book on track, rewritten sentences, and critically questioned them at a speed that is second to none, what a blessing. You are and have been my joker or the ace up my sleeve.

Maren Schelly

Contents

About the Authors

Maren Schelly, born on 11.05.1976, is a certified pediatric nurse (since 1998), practice instructor (since 2000), and urotherapist (since 2009). Until the end of 1999, she worked on the children's ward at the state hospital in Bregenz/Austria. After that, she began her work at the Wilhelmstift Children's Hospital, Hamburg, where she first worked on the children's infection ward and then from 2003 to 2019 as a pediatric nurse and practice instructor on a children's ward with a focus on hand surgery, surgery, facial surgery, burn surgery, and orthopedics, from 2012 as deputy ward manager. In 2012, she began working part-time in the malformation consultation hour of pediatric hand surgery, burn and facial surgery, which became a full-time position in 2019. Since 2015, she has been giving lectures at national and international hand surgery congresses.

Anna-Lena Dunse, born on 09.01.1991, completed her training as an occupational therapist in 2009 and subsequently worked in various practices in the pediatric field. In 2014, she underwent further training in sensory integration therapy and in 2017 successfully completed her certification as a hand therapist at the AfH. In addition to her work in the pediatric field, after her graduation as a hand therapist, she gained experience in treating patients with acute and chronic orthopedic and hand surgical diseases or injuries. Since 2018, she has been working at the Wilhelmstift Children's Hospital in the Department of Hand Surgery with a focus on malformation surgery. The focus is on the treatment of children and adolescents before and after surgical procedures. Since 2022, she has also been working part-time in the Department of Neonatology.

Development of the Hand

1

Contents

The hand, with its magnificent motor and receptive ability, plays a crucial role in human development. Almost nowhere else are tactile bodies located in such high density, which is disproportionately reflected in the representation of the sensory hand areas in the cerebrum. The touch senses of the hands are of crucial importance in the maturation and learning process. Self-perception, which informs the brain at all times about the position of the hand and fingers in space and about the direction and speed, is one of the most important prerequisites for the development of motor skills. The connection of the highly sensitive sense of touch with motor precision makes the hand the most significant tactile tool of humans. The close interaction between hand and brain becomes apparent in sign language communication, the execution of delicate activities, the palpation of objects, the ability to make isolated movements of individual fingers, and through the high speed of movement (Wehr and Weinmann 2005). The ability to compensate for individual gripping functions by reorientation also shows the flexible relationship between hand and brain.

It is astonishing how quickly a "newly" developed finger position is represented in the cortical field of the brain, which develops in early childhood within a few weeks (e.g., after pollicization/ Chap. 3). The neuronal basis of these changes is not yet fully understood. It is suspected that new connections in the synaptic interconnections are formed by performing altered movement sequences (Wehr and Weinmann 2005). This functional reorientation after surgical interventions and/or therapeutic measures is an excellent example of the flexible relationship between hand and nervous system. Our possibilities in therapy are based on this interaction. Visuomotorics, the coordination of visual perception and movement, allows us to achieve therapeutic successes by practicing eye-hand coordination. Therefore, both the anatomy and the motor skills and self-perception of the patient must be taken into account during the entire treatment.

The **hand therapeutic care of infants and toddlers with congenital hand malformations** is a highly specialized, constantly evolving field. The anatomical changes, rapid growth, and

development of children pose great challenges
to us as therapists. At the same time, the delicate, elastic tissue and the rapid learning ability
of the child's brain provide an optimal prerequisite for successful therapy. An improvement
in the gripping function in infancy and early
childhood promotes the child's development
and stimulates the interaction between hand and
brain. Through early, regular manual therapy
and constant splinting in infancy and early childhood, the gripping function can be improved
and in some cases fully restored. The results
after surgical corrections are maintained and
improved by these measures. Since many malformations lack essential structures (Fig. 1.1),
even surgery cannot build a normal-looking
hand with full function. The goal is to create and
maintain the best possible hand function to enable the child to lead an independent life.

For successful therapy and development,
each child must be accompanied holistically by
an interdisciplinary team. An individually tai-
lored therapy concept is created together with
the child and the parents and is continuously
adapted during growth, taking into account the
child's development. The focus is not only on
the body structures and gripping functions,
but also on the child's participation in his individual everyday life and his environment. The
bio-psycho-social model according to ICF
(International Classification of Functioning,
Disability and Health) provides a good structure
for this.

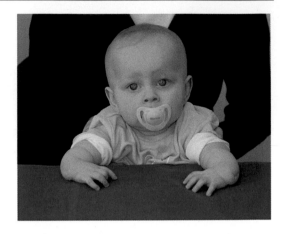

Fig. 1.1 9-month-old boy with radial longitudinal
reduction defect (radial club hand), thumb aplasia and
finger flexion contractures on both sides (Chap. 2). ©
Children's Hospital Wilhelmstift, with kind permission

In order to help the little patients, a high understanding of the healthy as well as malformation-
specific anatomical pathology and physiology is
required. Knowledge of the motor and receptive
possibilities of the healthy child in the various
developmental phases allows conclusions to be
drawn about the need for intervention in a malformed child. The sensory systems are included
in the therapies and the ability to perceive senses
and to react to them is taken into account in the
care. For example, an infant should be given
enough time for unhindered gripping during
splint therapy in order to experience himself and
his environment and thus further develop both
motor and receptive skills.

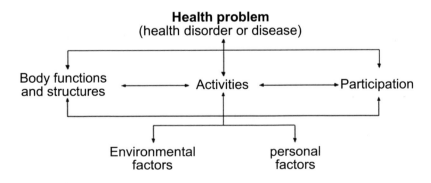

The bio-psycho-social model. (Source: https://www.bfarm.de/DE/Kodiersysteme/Klassifikationen/ICF/_node.html6,
with kind permission)

Table 1.1 Definition of age groups—National Association of Statutory Health Insurance Physicians (Berlin as of 04.2021)

Definition of age groups	
Newborn	Until the completed 28th day of life
Infant	Until the completed 12th month of life
Toddler	Until the completed 3rd year of life
Child	Until the completed 12th year of life
Teenager	Until the completed 18th year of life

In this first chapter, after a brief description of the prenatal development of the upper extremity and the formation of congenital anomalies, the postnatal development follows. The postnatal development initially refers to the bony development in growth. This is followed by the anatomy and physiology of the upper extremities. After the nerve supply, we turn to the gripping functions, graphomotor skills, and sensory systems, and conclude with the developmental phases from infancy to the 7th year of life.

In order to provide a clear classification for the age groups from newborn to teenager, we adhere to the definition of the National Association of Statutory Health Insurance Physicians (Table 1.1).

1.1 Prenatal Development of the Hand

The development of the hand predominantly takes place in the first weeks of pregnancy. Congenital anomalies largely occur during this early phase (Table 1.2).

▶ ***Apoptosis** is a form of programmed cell death. During embryonic development, the separation of the fingers occurs through apoptosis. In the 5th week after fertilization, the arm bud is paddle-shaped, the fingers are still connected. The interdigital cell death separates the fingers from each other. The affected cells die without damaging the neighboring cells.

Malformations of the upper extremities can be caused by genetic factors, environmental influences, or syndromal diseases. However, most causes of congenital (=inborn) malformations are still unknown. The OMT classification divides congenital anomalies into malformations, deformations, and dysplasias (Table 1.3).

1.2 Postnatal Development of the Hand

From a biomechanical point of view, the hand is certainly the most complicated part of the body. Including the ulna and radius, the hand consists of 29 individual bones. These are connected by a complicated system of ligaments and tendons.

1.2.1 Bone Development

In the first years of life, the ends of the bones and the carpal bones are still cartilaginous. Therefore, the joint spaces are not delineated on X-rays and thus not visible (Fig. 1.2). This makes the evaluation of X-rays in the first years of life difficult. In addition, the bone development of the malformed extremity is usually delayed compared to normal skeletal development.

In the carpus, the bone core of the capitate bone (Os capitatum) becomes visible first (Fig. 1.2) (Strassmair et al. 2009) followed by the hamate bone (Os hamatum) and gradually the other carpal bones. The pisiform bone (Os pisiforme) is the last to become visible (Fig. 1.3). The complete ossification of the scaphoid bone (Os scaphoideum) takes the longest. Only at the age of 14 are all structures of the carpal bones fully visible. The entire ossification is completed at about 15 years of age (Marzi 2006). The length growth of the bones occurs via the growth plates, which contribute to varying degrees. The humerus grows 80% proximally and 20% distally. The ratio is reversed for the ulna (Ulna) and the radius (Radius) (Marzi 2006). The growth plates close during puberty between the ages of 14 and 18.

Table 1.2 Prenatal development of the upper extremity

Prenatal development of the upper extremity *(Bommbas-Ebert et al. 2011)*

Embryonic stage/ Day after fertilization of the egg cell	Developmental steps
12 approx. 30 days	Buds of the upper extremity form
14 approx. 33 days	Formation of the hand plate
16 approx. 39 days	Upper and lower arm bones form cartilaginously, the shoulder joint develops
17 approx. 42–44 days	Metacarpal rays form cartilaginously
18 approx. 44–48 days	Proximal phalanges form cartilaginously
19 approx. 48–51 days	Middle phalanges form cartilaginously, apoptosis* begins
20 approx. 51–53 days	The distal phalanges form cartilaginously, apoptosis progresses
22 approx. 54–56 days	Ossification of the humerus, apoptosis is completed
23 approx. 56–60 days	Ossification of the phalanges

Table 1.3 OMT Classification

OMT Classification

Congenital anomalies are divided into malformations, deformations, and dysplasias in the internationally recognized OMT classification (Oberg et al. 2015)

Origin of congenital anomalies

Malformations	3.5 to the 8th GW (=gestational week) • e.g. clubhand (Chap. 2), thumb hypoplasia and aplasia (Chap. 3)
Deformations	act externally on the fetus. They can occur throughout the entire pregnancy • e.g. constriction ring syndrome
Dysplasias	3.5 to the 5th GW • e.g. thumb-in-palm deformity, arthrogryposis (Chap. 4), macrodactyly, osteochondromas Dysplasias show up at different times: Macrodactylies at birth, osteochondromas in the first years of life, congenital tumors also later. The structures are already present in utero

1.2.2 Anatomy and Grasping Functions

1.2.2.1 Thumb

The thumb (Digitus I) plays a key role in the hand due to its diverse range of motion.

The uniqueness of thumb function is due to the morphology of the joints and a high number of muscles. The opposition movement is used most frequently. In this movement, the thumb approaches the other fingers.

The thumb has only two phalanges:
the distal phalanx and
the proximal phalanx.

The thumb ray includes the saddle joint and the first metacarpal bone and consists of:

- the saddle joint (carpometacarpal joint/CMC) between the trapezium (Os trapezium) and the first metacarpal bone (Os metacarpale I),
- the base joint (metacarpophalangeal joint/ MCP I) between the first metacarpal bone and the proximal phalanx,
- the end joint (interphalangeal joint/IP) between the proximal and the distal phalanx.

1.2.2.2 Fingers

Fingers II–V (Digitus II–V) each consist of three phalanges, the proximal phalanx, the medial phalanx, and the distal phalanx, with three joints each:

- the metacarpophalangeal joints (MCP II-V) between the metacarpal bones and the proximal phalanges,

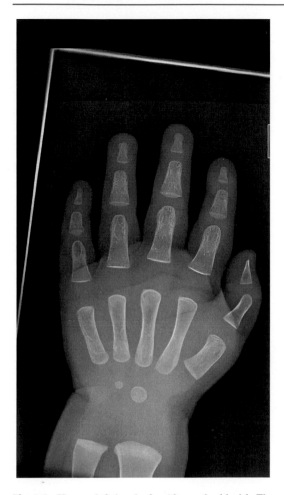

Fig. 1.2 X-ray—left hand of a 10-month-old girl. The joint spaces are not yet radiologically delineated due to the still cartilaginous ends of the adjacent limbs. The bone cores of the capitate bone and the hamate bone are visible. (© Children's Hospital Wilhelmstift, with kind permission)

- the middle joints (proximal interphalangeal joints/PIP II–V) between the proximal and the medial phalanges,
- and the end joints (distal interphalangeal joints/DIP II–V) between the medial and the distal phalanges.

Each finger forms a finger ray with its respective metacarpal bone, which forms the connection to the carpus.

The following dynamic sequences of movement are important for a good gripping function of the hand:

- The large fist:
  The base, middle, and end joints are bent, the fingertips touch the flexion groove of the palm (Fig. 1.4a).
- The small fist:
  The base joints are extended, the middle and end joints are bent, there is no cavity visible between the finger joints (Fig. 1.4b).
- The lumbrical grip:
  The base joints are bent, the middle and end joints are extended (Fig. 1.4c).
- The opposition:
  The thumb is opposite fingers II–V. It is measured according to the Kapandji index (Figs. 1.4d and 1.6a–c).
- Maximum hand span:
  When the fingers are spread apart, the hand flattens and achieves the greatest distance between the little finger and thumb tip, the so-called hand span (Fig. 1.4e).

Directions of movement of the finger joints
The thumb saddle joint is special because it has two degrees of freedom, which are

- Abduction and adduction
- Palmar flexion and retropulsion (= maximum dorsal extension)
  as well as a combination movement
- The opposition.

The base joints of the thumb and fingers II–V are ellipsoid joints, which can perform the movements:

- Extension and flexion
- Abduction and adduction.

The end joint of the thumb and the middle and end joints of fingers II–V are hinge joints, which can perform the movements:

- Extension and flexion.

Ranges of Motion of the Finger Joints
(These are average values – there are large normal variations)

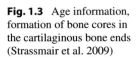

Fig. 1.3 Age information, formation of bone cores in the cartilaginous bone ends (Strassmair et al. 2009)

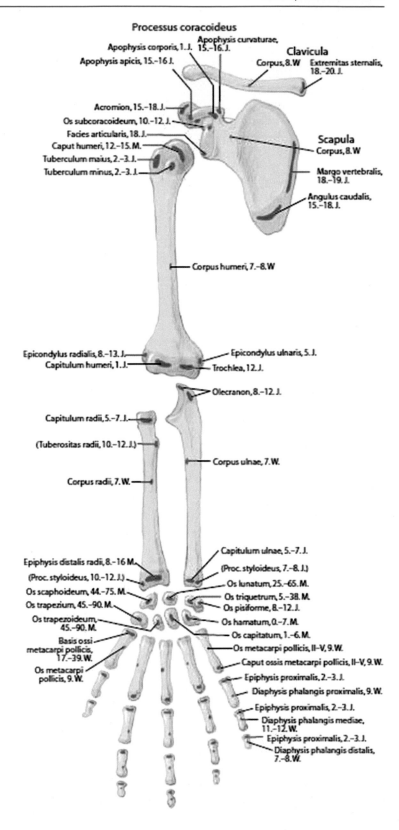

Processus coracoideus
Apophysis curvaturae, 15.–16. J.
Apophysis corporis, 1. J.
Apophysis apicis, 15.–16 J.

Clavicula
Corpus, 8. W   Extremitas sternalis, 18.–20. J.

Acromion, 15.–18. J.
Os subcoracoideum, 10.–12. J.
Facies articularis, 18. J.
Caput humeri, 12.–15. M.
Tuberculum maius, 2.–3. J.
Tuberculum minus, 2.–3. J.

Scapula
Corpus, 8. W

Margo vertebralis, 18.–19. J.

Angulus caudalis, 15.–18. J.

Corpus humeri, 7.–8. W

Epicondylus radialis, 8.–13. J.
Capitulum humeri, 1. J.

Epicondylus ulnaris, 5. J.
Trochlea, 12. J.

Olecranon, 8.–12. J.

Capitulum radii, 5.–7. J.

(Tuberositas radii, 10.–12. J.)

Corpus ulnae, 7. W.

Corpus radii, 7. W.

Capitulum ulnae, 5.–7. J.

Epiphysis distalis radii, 8.–16 M.
(Proc. styloideus, 10.–12. J.)
Os scaphoideum, 44.–75. M.
Os trapezium, 45.–90. M.
Os trapezoideum, 45.–90. M.
Basis ossi metacarpi pollicis, 17.–39. W.
Os metacarpi pollicis, 9. W.

(Proc. styloideus, 7.–8. J.)
Os lunatum, 25.–65. M.
Os triquetrum, 5.–38. M.
Os pisiforme, 8.–12. J.
Os hamatum, 0.–7. M.
Os capitatum, 1.–6. M.
Os metacarpi pollicis, II–V, 9. W.
Caput ossis metacarpi pollicis, II–V, 9. W.
Epiphysis proximalis, 2.–3. J.
Diaphysis phalangis proximalis, 9. W.
Epiphysis proximalis, 2.–3. J.
Diaphysis phalangis mediae, 11.–12. W.
Epiphysis proximalis, 2.–3. J.
Diaphysis phalangis distalis, 7.–8. W.

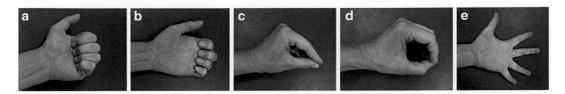

Fig. 1.4 a Large fist, **b** Small fist, **c** Lumbrical grip, **d** Opposition, **e** Maximum hand span. (© Kinderkrankenhaus Wilhelmstift, with kind permission)

Metacarpophalangeal joints of fingers II–V:

- Flexion 90°
- Extension 40°
- Abduction 15°
- Adduction 15°

Metacarpophalangeal joint of the thumb:

- Flexion 80°
- Extension 0°
- slight abduction and adduction

Proximal interphalangeal joints of fingers II–V:

- Flexion 130°
- Extension 0°

Distal interphalangeal joints of fingers I–V:

- Flexion 90°
- Extension 30° (Zumhasch et al. 2012).

Saddle joint:

In adduction, the thumb lies against the 2nd metacarpal bone. This is the 0° position. The thumb spreading is divided into a palmar abduction (up to 45°) (Fig. 1.5a) and a radial abduction (up to 60°) (Fig. 1.5b) (Zumhasch et al. 2012). The retroversion (also called retropulsion) describes the maximum active extension of the thumb ray beyond the plane of the hand.

Quick Movement Checks

A quick method to check the mobility of fingers II–V is for flexion:

- performing the small and large fist

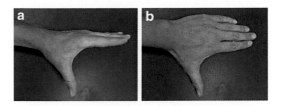

Fig. 1.5 a Palmar abduction, **b** Radial abduction. (© Children's Hospital Wilhelmstift, with kind permission)

and for extension:

- opening the hand. The hand lies with the back of the hand on the table and the fingernails touch the surface.

If a finger cannot fully perform the small or large fist, the range of motion of the base, middle, and end joint are measured, as well as the fingertip-palm distance (FKHA). The distance between the fingertip and the palm crease is measured in cm. If full extension is not possible, in addition to the movement measures, the fingernail-table distance (FNTA) is also recorded, with the back of the hand lying on the table. The distance between the fingernail and the table is measured in cm. To capture the overall mobility (the opposition) of the thumb ray, the Kapandji index is a simple and reliable method. The thumb tip touches the following finger areas (Fig. 1.6a–c). If the 6, the tip of the little finger, is reached, the thumb is in maximum palmar adduction (Fig. 1.6b).

When touching the 10 (distal palm crease), in addition to the saddle joint, the base and the end joint are also bent (Fig. 1.6c). All joints of the thumb ray are free and very mobile.

The test is only meaningful if the thumb forms an arc, i.e., there is a distance between the

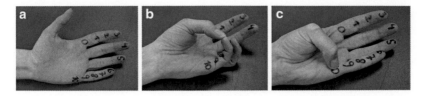

Fig. 1.6 **a** Measurement points of the Kapandji index, by definition, starting with 0, **b** maximum palmar abduction of the thumb **c** maximum flexion of the thumb. (© Children's Hospital Wilhelmstift, with kind permission)

thumb and the palm of the hand. If the thumb is only placed in the palm, the 10 can be reached, but the test is worthless (Kapandji 2016). This can be observed in the thumb-in-palm deformity. The thumb lies in the palm, but cannot or only insufficiently be actively brought into abduction and extension (Fig. 1.7) (Chap. 5).

The retroversion of the thumb is determined by spreading it radially in the plane and lifting it dorsally. After a pollicization (= index finger converted into the thumb position) (Chap. 3), the retroversion is not feasible. If the thumb is severely hypoplastic or not present, the opposition movement cannot be performed in any way. In some cases, the flexion and extension of fingers 2–5 are also insufficient. The pinch grip, also known as the side grip or interdigital grip, becomes the dominant form of grip in this case. The children move their fingers in abduction and adduction to hold and guide objects (Fig. 1.8) (Chaps. 2, 3 and 5).

1.2.2.3 Ligamentous Capsule Apparatus

In order to perform both delicate tasks and to grip powerfully, a sophisticated movement

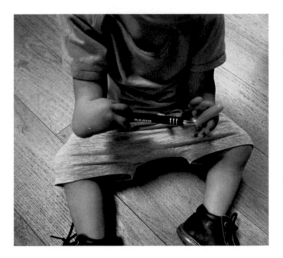

Fig. 1.8 18-month-old boy with bilateral radial longitudinal reduction defect (RLD), thumb aplasia on the right, thumb hypoplasia on the left, and finger flexion contractures on both sides. Due to the missing or hypoplastic thumbs and the insufficient flexion and extension of the fingers, the interdigital grip has become the dominant form of grip. (© Children's Hospital Wilhelmstift, with kind permission)

apparatus consisting of bones, muscles, countless ligaments, and tendons is required. The **ligamentous capsule apparatus** is responsible for stabilizing the joints. At the same time, it centers the extensors and flexors during movement. The deep and superficial collateral ligaments, together with the palmar and dorsal connective tissue plate, maintain joint surface contact. This ensures a high stability of the joints during movement (Fig. 1.9) (Kapandji 2016). In children with arthrogryposis-like diseases, there may be hypermobility of the basic and middle joints into hyperextension (Chap. 5). This is primarily due to instability of the palmar plate. A characteristic of hypermobile joints is the retracted skin on the dorsal side over the middle

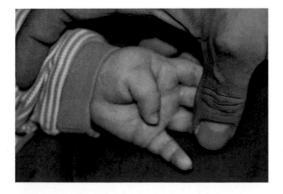

Fig. 1.7 10-week-old boy with a thumb-in-palm deformity. (© Children's Hospital Wilhelmstift, with kind permission)

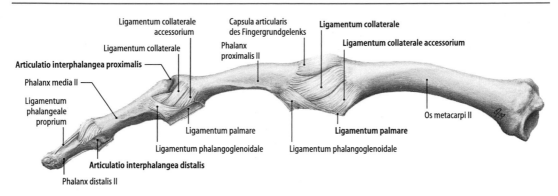

Fig. 1.9 Ligamentous capsule apparatus of an index finger (Atlas of Human Anatomy, Tillmann 2020)

joints (Fig. 1.10). Dysfunctions of the band-like structures are also evident in thumb hypoplasia (Chap. 3).

1.2.2.4 Flexor Tendon Apparatus
The flexor tendon apparatus consists of the flexor tendons with their tendon sheaths, and the annular and cruciate ligaments. The annular and cruciate ligaments have the task of centering and guiding the flexor tendon sheath on the finger skeleton, thus ensuring the sliding of the tendons in the tendon sheath close to the bone. The annular and cruciate ligaments contract accordion-like during flexion and glide apart during extension (Fig. 1.11).

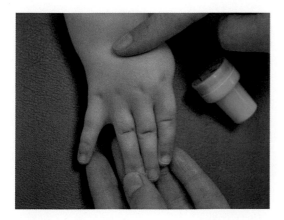

Fig. 1.10 22-month-old girl with Sheldon-Hall syndrome (Chap. 5). The middle joints of fingers II-IV tend to hyperextend, forming retractions on the dorsal skin side. (© Children's Hospital Wilhelmstift, with kind permission)

1.2.2.5 Extensor Apparatus
The extensor apparatus consists of the extensor tendons, which extend from the back of the hand into the dorsal aponeurosis. The dorsal aponeurosis is a triangularly structured connective tissue plate located on the dorsal side of the finger. The interossei, the lumbricals, as well as the tendon fibers of the M. extensor digitorum, the M. extensor indicis, and the M extensor digiti minimi attach to it. Together, they form this structure and perform precise extensions of the middle and end joints as well as a flexion of the base joints (Figs. 1.11, 1.14 and 1.15) (Schmidt and Lanz 2003). Incorrectly inserted lumbricals and/or a weakened dorsal aponeurosis can be causes of camptodactyly (Chap. 4). The tendons of the M. extensor digitorum (Fig. 1.11) run dorsally over the base joints. Their tendency to deviate towards the ulnar side is limited by the **radial extensor hood** (Fig. 1.12). The situation is different in the case of arthrogryposis-like diseases. In some cases, a clear ulnar deviation in the base joints of fingers II-V can be seen (the so-called windblown hand deformity) (Fig. 1.13) (Chap. 5).

1.2.2.6 Extrinsic Musculature
In the hand, intrinsic and extrinsic muscles ensure a perfect interplay of muscles and tendons. The hand has 33 muscles. A large part of them are located in the forearm, the so-called extrinsic musculature, whose tendons extend into the hand (Table 1.4).

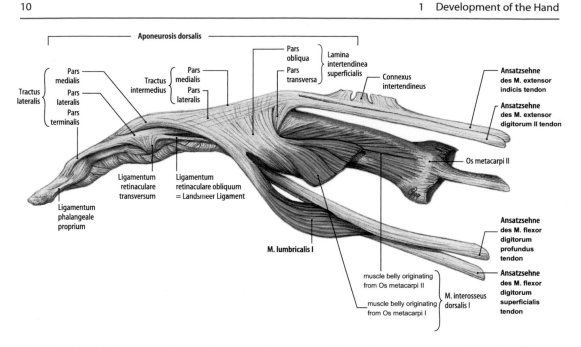

Fig. 1.11 The dorsal aponeurosis, muscles, and tendons of the right index finger, view from radial (Atlas of Human Anatomy, Tillmann 2020)

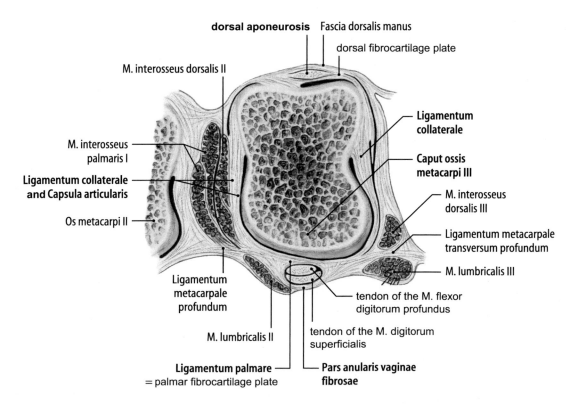

Fig. 1.12 Cross-section through the base joint of the middle finger. View of the distal cut surface. (Atlas of Human Anatomy, Tillmann 2020)

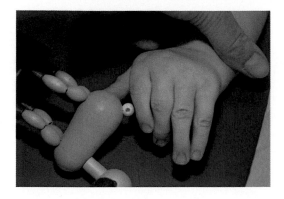

Fig. 1.13 One-year-old boy with a distal arthrogryposis, there is a windblown hand deformity of fingers II–V and a thumb-in-palm deformity. (© Children's Hospital Wilhelmstift, with kind permission)

▶ The extrinsic muscles originate outside the hand, cross, move and stabilize the wrist, and attach in the hand.

1.2.2.7 Pronators and Supinators

The following muscles are primarily responsible for the execution of pronation and supination in the distal and proximal radioulnar joint (Table 1.5):

1.2.2.8 Intrinsic Musculature

The intrinsic musculature is formed from the thenar on the thumb side and the hypothenar on the little finger side. Other small muscles lie between the metacarpal bones (Table 1.6).

▶ The intrinsic muscles have their origin and insertion in the hand.

The diverse movements and the harmonious interplay between the intrinsic and extrinsic muscles are referred to as synergy.

1.2.2.9 Synergistic Effect

The **synergistic effect** is clearly visible in the example of a powerful fist closure. When the wrist is extended, the fingers are automatically flexed. When the wrist is flexed, the fingers automatically extend. The fingers can be flexed in wrist flexion, but the fist closure is powerless. The wrist extensors work synergistically with the long finger flexors. The flexors in the

wrist work synergistically with the long finger extensors (Kapandji 2016). In order to perform movements, a harmonious interplay between opposing muscles must take place, the so-called agonists and antagonists. The movements of the biceps and triceps illustrate this. When the agonist, the biceps, contracts to bend the elbow, the antagonist, the triceps, must allow the movement by stretching. When the elbow is extended, the triceps is the agonist and the biceps is the antagonist, allowing the extension by stretching. If the musculature of the hand and forearm is hypotrophic or hypoplastic, a dysbalance of the pulling forces occurs. The agonists and antagonists cannot work harmoniously and the synergistic effect is significantly restricted (Chaps. 2–5). The fingers and the wrist lose a large part of their function, their strength and their skill. If left untreated, contractures can develop or intensify due to the imbalances. The leverage changes. The function is further restricted.

1.2.2.10 Wrist

The range of motion of the **wrist** allows the hand to assume an optimal gripping position. Together with the pro- and supination of the forearm as well as the elbow and shoulder mobility, the hand can grip and hold at any conceivable angle.

The following joints are involved in the movement of the wrist:

- Between radius/ulna and carpus (Articulatio Radiocarpalis)
- Between proximal and distal row of carpal bones (Articulatio Mediocarpalis)

The carpus, which consists of eight small bones, is an ellipsoid joint that allows the degrees of freedom:

- Extension/Flexion and
- Radial- / Ulnar deviation.

Circumduction is a combination of the four movements.

The healthy wrist exhibits:
an extension of approx. 85°,

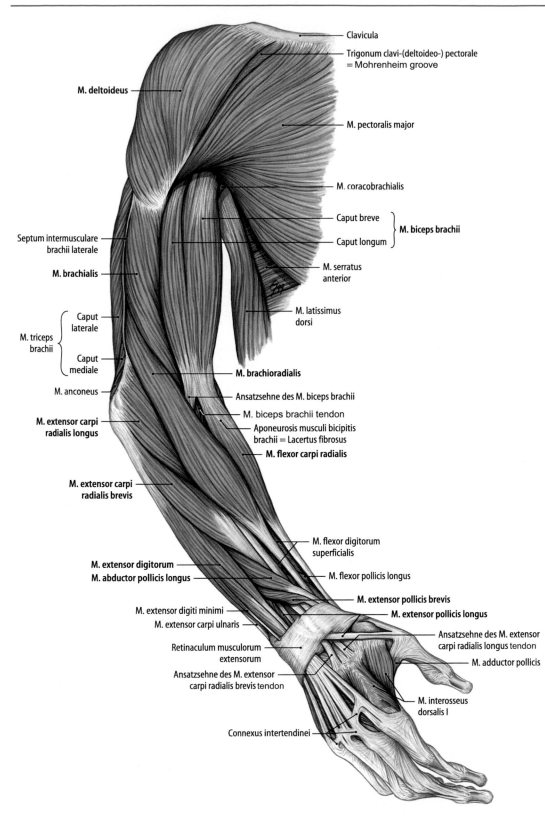

Fig. 1.14 Muscles of the right arm, slight flexion in the elbow, indication of a pronation (Atlas of Human Anatomy, Tillmann 2020)

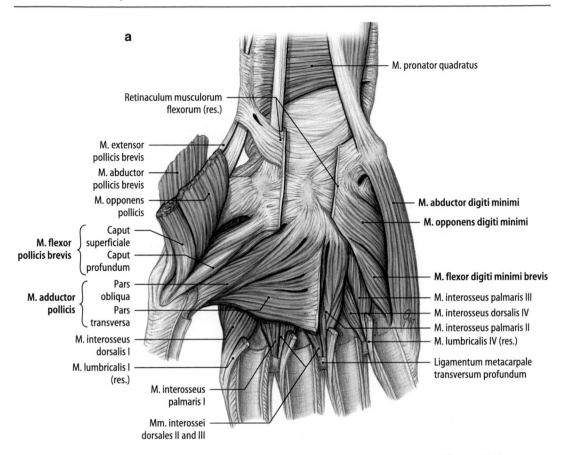

Fig. 1.15 Intrinsic muscles of the right hand, view from palmar (Atlas of Human Anatomy, Tillmann 2020)

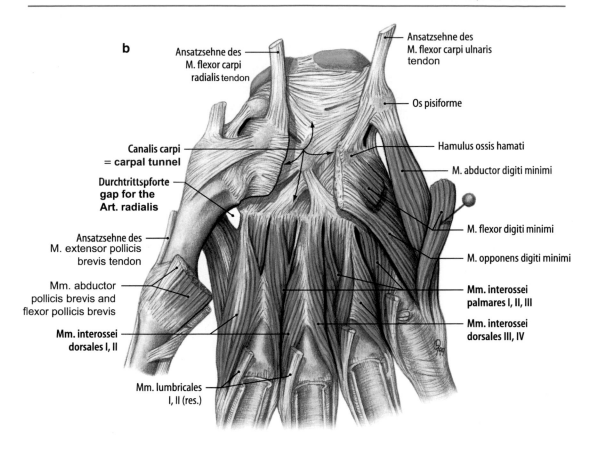

b

Ansatzsehne des
M. flexor carpi
radialis tendon

Ansatzsehne des
M. flexor carpi ulnaris
tendon

Os pisiforme

Canalis carpi
= carpal tunnel

Hamulus ossis hamati

M. abductor digiti minimi

Durchtrittspforte
gap for the
Art. radialis

Ansatzsehne des
M. extensor pollicis
brevis tendon

M. flexor digiti minimi

M. opponens digiti minimi

Mm. abductor
pollicis brevis and
flexor pollicis brevis

Mm. interossei
palmares I, II, III

Mm. interossei
dorsales I, II

Mm. interossei
dorsales III, IV

Mm. lumbricales
I, II (res.)

Fig. 1.15 (continued)

a flexion of approx. 85°,

an ulnar deviation of approx. 45° (bending towards the little finger)

and a radial deviation of approx. 15° (bending towards the thumb).

Both passive extension and passive flexion are greater in pronation than in supination (Kapandji 2016). The fingers have an optimal efficiency when the wrist is in approx. 30–40° extension and 15° ulnar deviation. In this position, the finger flexors can develop their full strength. The range of motion of the hand is all the smaller, the less the wrist can be moved due to contractures or underdeveloped or missing muscles. A stronger ulnar deviation already significantly reduces the strength of the fingers, which can be observed in arthrogryposis-like diseases (Fig. 1.16) (Chap. 5).

Good stability in the wrist is a prerequisite for differentiated finger mobility. If the wrist is in a malposition, compensatory movements occur from the shoulder and elbow. These movements are less differentiated in their coordination and accuracy. Children often complain of pain when writing for a long time.

▶ For many gripping functions, the optimal, powerful wrist position is an extension of approx. 30–40° and an ulnar deviation of approx.15°

1.2.2.11 Forearm

The **forearm** consists of two bones, the ulna and the radius. The rotation of the forearm occurs between these two bones in the distal and proximal radioulnar joint and allows the hand a high range of motion with a large

Table 1.4 Extrinsic Musculature

Extrinsic Musculature	
• Extensor Muscles:	
M.extensor carpi ulnaris (ECU)	Its main task is ulnar deviation and the guidance of the supination movement, it is involved in pressure regulation in the carpus and is the most important wrist stabilizer
M.extensor carpi radialis longus (ECRL)	Is responsible for dorsal extension and radial deviation
M. extensor carpi radialis brevis (ECRB)	Is responsible for dorsal extension in the wrist
M.extensor digitorum communis (EDC)	Is responsible for the extension of fingers II-V and involved in dorsal extension and ulnar deviation of the wrist
M. extensor indicis proprius (EIP)	Is responsible for the isolated extension of the index finger
M extensor digiti minimi (EDM)	Is responsible for the extension and abduction of the little finger and involved in ulnar deviation and dorsal extension of the wrist
M. abductor pollicis longus (APL)	Stabilizes the saddle joint and abducts the thumb
M. extensor pollicis brevis (EPB)	Is responsible for the extension and abduction of the thumb's metacarpophalangeal joint
M. extensor pollicis longus (EPL)	Is responsible for the extension and abduction of the thumb and involved in radial deviation and dorsal extension of the wrist
• Flexor Muscles:	
M. flexor carpi ulnaris (FCU)	Is responsible for palmar flexion and involved in ulnar deviation
M. flexor carpi radialis (FCR)	Is responsible for palmar flexion, stabilization of the carpus, and centering of the carpal bones during radial deviation
M. flexor digitorum superficialis (FDS)	Is responsible for the flexion of the proximal and middle joints and supports palmar flexion in the wrist
M. flexor digitorum profundus (FDP)	Is responsible for the flexion of fingers II-V in the proximal, middle, and distal joints and supports palmar flexion in the wrist
M. flexor pollicis longus (FPL)	Is responsible for the flexion of all thumb joints

Table 1.5 Musculature for Pronation and Supination

Pronators and Supinators	
• Pronators	
M. pronator teres	Strong two-headed muscle in the proximal forearm (Caput humerale/Caput ulnare). It performs pronation in the forearm and is slightly involved in the flexion of the elbow
M. pronator quadratus	Runs in the distal forearm, is the most important pronator and stabilizes the distal radioulnar joint
• Supinators	
M. biceps brachii	No supinatory effect when the elbow is extended, the supination increases with increasing elbow flexion
M. supinator	Most important muscle for performing supination in any functional position of the elbow joint

gripping accuracy. The interosseous membrane of the forearm (Membrana interossea antebrachii) allows the displacement of the ulna and radius during movements and simultaneously secures the mechanical coupling. Since the rotation movement in most cases occurs together with the shoulder, to determine the complete pronation and supination, the forearm must lie against the body and the elbow joint must be bent by 90°. In the supination position, the palm of the hand faces cranially (upwards) and the thumb laterally (outwards). The radius and ulna are parallel to each other. In the pronation position, the palm of the hand faces caudally (downwards) and the thumb medially (inwards). The radius crosses over the ulna. In the neutral-zero position, the thumb points cranially. From this position, the degrees of

Table 1.6 Intrinsic Musculature

Intrinsic Musculature	
• Thenar muscles:	
M. adductor pollicis	The strongest muscle of the hand. It adducts the thumb and supports the opposition
M. opponens pollicis	Is responsible for the opposition and supports the adduction
M. abductor pollicis brevis	Is responsible for the abduction of the thumb
M. flexor pollicis brevis	Is responsible for the flexion mainly in the thumb base joint
• Hypothenar muscles:	
M. abductor digiti minimi	Abducts the little finger
M. flexor digiti minimi	Is responsible for the flexion of the little finger base joint
M. opponens digiti minimi	Is responsible for the opposition movement of the little finger
• Lumbrical muscles:	
Mm. lumbricales	Are four short hand muscles, responsible for the flexion of the finger base joints II-V and for the extension in the middle and end joints of the fingers II-V, they originate from the tendons of the M. extensor Profundus
• Interosseous muscles:	
Mm. interossei palmares Mm. interossei dorsales	The three muscles are responsible for the adduction of fingers II, IV, V to the middle finger, for the flexion in the base joints II, IV, V as well as the extension in the middle and end joints of the fingers II, IV and V, they radiate into the extensor aponeurosis The four muscles are responsible for the flexion in the base joints II-IV as well as the extension in the middle and end joints of the fingers II–IV, they also perform the abduction from the middle finger, they radiate into the extensor aponeurosis

movement are measured. In a healthy person, pronation is approximately 85° and supination is approximately 90° (Kapandji 2016). If the shoulder joint is involved in the movement, a complete rotation of 360° can occur with the arm hanging down.

Pronation and supination allow the hand to make quick, precise, and powerful movements. If supination and pronation cannot be performed due to a missing radius, a compensatory movement occurs from the shoulder and the entire upper body. This movement is less powerful, inefficient, and slower, and the range of motion is significantly restricted (Fig. 1.17) (Chap. 2).

1.2.2.12 Elbow Joint

The **elbow joint** consists of three partial joints and connects the humerus (Humerus) with the forearm bones.

It is composed of the following joints:

- Between the humerus and ulna (Articulatio humeroulnaris)
- Between the humerus and radius (Articulatio humeroradialis)

- Between the radius and ulna (Articulatio radioulnaris proximalis)

It has two axes of movement:

- Flexion and extension between the humerus and ulna
- Pronation and supination in the proximal radioulnar joint.

For the range of motion of the elbow, extension and flexion are measured. A healthy elbow has a maximum flexion of 140°. Children, especially girls, can often hyperextend by 20°. Through the flexion of the elbow joint, the hand effortlessly reaches the shoulder and mouth. With the help of pronation and supination, a fork can be brought to and away from the mouth. Including the shoulder, the hair can be combed or a backpack can be put on. The mobility of the elbow favors a persistent, clean writing flow. It is indispensable for food intake. Stiff elbow joints in extension prevent independent food intake, which is the case in children with arthrogryposis with extension contractures (Chap. 5).

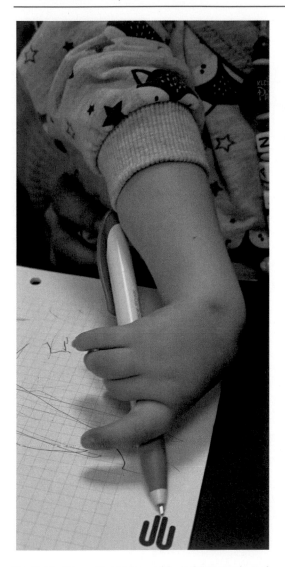

Fig. 1.16 18-month-old boy with Arthrogryposis multiplex congenita (AMC). There is a clear malposition of the wrist in flexion and ulnar deviation, the graphomotor skills are significantly impaired. (© Children's Hospital Wilhelmstift, with kind permission)

Food intake is only possible with a stiff or non-existent elbow joint if the arm is very short (Fig. 1.18) (TAR syndrome/Chap. 2). Therefore, it is important to always align the focus of treatment and surgical interventions with the given gripping function in order not to disturb useful replacement grips.

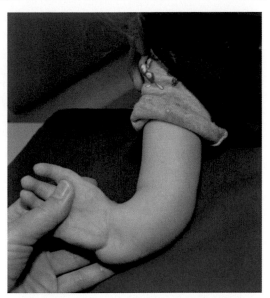

Fig. 1.17 2-year-old boy with radial longitudinal reduction defect (= radial club hand). To allow the palm to point cranially, the arm must be rotated from the shoulder and body. (© Children's Hospital Wilhelmstift, with kind permission)

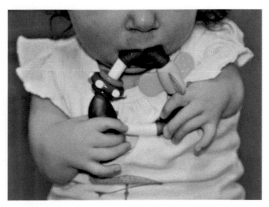

Fig. 1.18 16-month-old girl with TAR syndrome. Severely shortened arms, no developed elbow joint. Due to the shortness of the arms and bending of the wrists, the child can reach the mouth. Straightening the wrists would take away this important function. (© Children's Hospital Wilhelmstift, with kind permission)

1.2.2.13 Shoulder Joint
The **shoulder joint**, with its small joint socket and muscular stabilization, is the most mobile of all joints in the human body.

The following joints are involved in the movement of the shoulder joint:

- the Articulatio glenohumeralis—between the Cavitas glenoidalis and the Caput humeri,
- the Articulatio acromioclavicularis—between the Acromion and the Clavicula
- the Articulatio sternoclavicularis—between the Clavicula and the Sternum

The great mobility of the shoulder requires securing by ligaments and a comprehensive muscle apparatus.

It has three degrees of freedom, which are executed around three main axes:

- the Anteversion (from 90° elevation to 180°) and Retroversion in the sagittal plane,
- the Abduction (from 90° in combination with Scapula movement up to 150°) and Adduction in the frontal plane,
- the External and Internal rotation in the horizontal plane.

If shoulder mobility is restricted, the fine motor skills of the hand cannot develop adequately, as children up to the age of 2 years use the shoulder intensively for graphomotor exercises or fine motor actions.

Restrictions of the shoulder joints occur, among other things, in Arthrogryposis multiplex congenita (Fig. 1.19) and the radial longitudinal reduction defect (Chaps. 2 and 5).

1.2.2.14 Nerve Trunks of the Upper Limbs

In order to move muscles, perceive touch, and perform activities, both the innervation of the muscles and the sensory nerve supply of the tissue and skin must be intact.

The sensory and motor innervation of the hand is carried out via the main nerve trunks, the Nervus ulnaris, the Nervus medianus, and the Nervus radialis. They originate from the Plexus brachialis, which is formed from the spinal nerves C5-Th1 (Table 1.7) (Zumhasch et al. 2012). Other **nerve trunks of the upper**

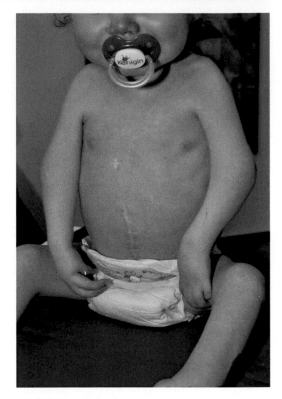

Fig. 1.19 17-month-old girl with a severe form of Arthrogryposis multiplex congenita without active shoulder mobility and with elbow stiffness in both arms. (© Children's Hospital Wilhelmstift, with kind permission)

Table 1.7 Nerves of the upper limbs

Nervus medianus	C8-Th1 (Th2)	Median nerve
Nervus ulnaris	C8-Th1 (Th2)	Ulnar nerve
Nervus radialis	C5-Th1	Radial nerve
Nervus axillaris	C5-Th1	Axillary nerve
Nervus musculocutaneus	C5-C7	Musculocutaneous nerve

limbs are the Nervus axillaris and the Nervus musculocutaneus.

▶ Innervation describes the neural supply of body tissues and organs (Pschyrembel 257).

An intact neural supply is indispensable for the development of grasping forms, graphomotor skills, and the expression of sensory systems.

1.2.3   Gripping Forms

The types of grip are described differently in the literature, we use the classification according to Waters and Bae (Waters and Bae 2012).

Overall, the types of grip are divided into two types:

- **Precision grip:** An object is manipulated between the fingertips.
- **Power or coarse grip:** An object is pressed by the long fingers against the thumb and thumb pad.

Precision or power grips can only be differentiated from the age of five. Good stability in the trunk and arm is important for good mobility in the hand. Therefore, both must be equally in focus during treatment.

1.2.3.1 Precision grips

Pincer grip, other terms are fine grip or tweezer grip. This precision grip requires good sensitivity and fine coordination. It is important for holding very small and fine objects, such as a thread, a pretzel stick or a lint. The thumb pad faces the index finger pad (Fig. 1.20a).

The **Penny grip** is a special form of the pincer grip (Neumann 1963) (Fig. 1.20b). It is used to pick up small objects. Objects like a coin can be picked up from a smooth surface using the fingernail.

The **Key grip** is also called lateral pincer grip or clamp grip. It is very powerful and stable and is used to turn a key in the lock or to open a

zipper. The object is pressed by the thumb pad against the radial side of the base or middle joint (Fig. 1.20c).

The **Three-point grip** is the most commonly used precision grip. This type of grip is also used to open bottles or pick up small objects (Fig. 1.20d). If the ring and little fingers are included, this grip form is extremely strong and stable.

1.2.3.2 Power or coarse grips

Coarse grip: All fingers are involved in gripping. They perform a flexion in all three joints. The bent thumb forms a counter bearing or lies over the bent fingers. All extrinsic and almost all intrinsic muscles are involved. This grip is used when holding a glass or operating a door handle (Fig. 1.21a).

Hook grip: The middle and end joints of all fingers are bent (Fig. 1.21b). This grip is used, for example, when carrying a bag.

1.2.3.3 Dynamic grips

The dynamic grips are combination grips of holding and moving during an action. The hand dynamically adapts during the manipulation, as when cutting, playing a string instrument, tying a bow, buttoning a coat. The thumb is involved in almost all grip forms and most power grips. The various grip forms are not or only partially executable for children with malformations. This becomes clear in the case of thumb aplasia and thumb hypoplasia (Chap. 3). In the case of a club hand, gripping is additionally complicated by a lack of mobility in the wrist and a restricted or missing pro- and supination (Chap. 2).

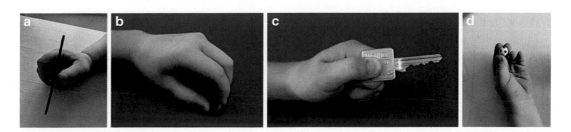

Fig. 1.20 **a** Pincer grip, **b** Penny grip, **c** Key grip, **d** Three-point grip. (© Children's Hospital Wilhelmstift, with kind permission)

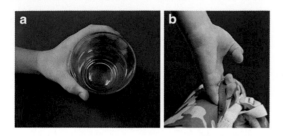

Fig. 1.21 a Power or coarse grip, **b** Hook grip. (© Children's Hospital Wilhelmstift, with kind permission)

> Children stand out by avoiding fine motor activities and quick frustration when performing these activities. In the case of restrictions due to underdeveloped or missing fingers, precision grips or power grips are not adequately possible. The implementation of pulling and pushing movements is jerky, uncoordinated and not very dynamic.

1.2.3.4 Lateral Pinch

The lateral pinch is also referred to as the interdigital grip or clamp grip. This type of grip is primarily used by people after amputation of the thumb or congenital severe thumb hypoplasia (Chaps. 2 and 3). Objects are grasped laterally between the index and middle fingers (Fig. 1.22).

1.2.3.5 In-Hand Manipulation

Complex dynamic movements, for example, are a prerequisite for physiological writing and can be examined in more detail based on the principle of in-hand manipulation.

Five movement patterns of in-hand manipulation are distinguished:

1. the translation (= displacement) from the fingertips to the palm, with or without stabilization,
2. the translation from the palm to the fingertips,
3. the simple rotation,
4. the complex rotation,
5. the shift movement.
   (Baumgarten and Strebel 2016).

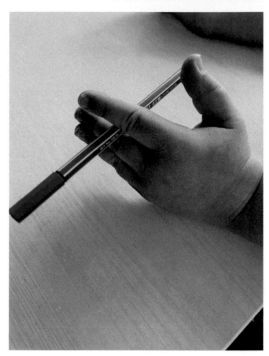

Fig. 1.22 Interdigital grip, lateral pinch (© Children's Hospital Wilhelmstift, with kind permission)

Examples:

1. The translation from the fingertips to the palm:
   A small stone is moved from the fingertip to the palm. The involved fingers move from extension to flexion for this.
2. With and without stabilization:
   An opposition is performed with the thumb and the index finger, while the remaining fingers stabilize and hold the small stone in the palm.
3. The translation from the palm to the fingertips:
   In contrast to the first movement, the thumb transports the stone from the palm to the fingertip. An isolated thumb movement is a prerequisite for this.
4. Simple rotation:
   Describes the rotation of the small stone with the fingertips by 90°. As when operating a spinning top or opening a twist cap.
5. The complex rotation:

A progression to the previous movement, where the small stone is rotated by 180°–360°. The fingers do not move as a unit, but isolated, as when turning a pen between the fingers.

6. The shift movement:
Linear displacement of a small object between MP and IP joints of fingers 2–5 with opposed and adducted thumb. For example, picking up a pen with one hand and moving it into the writing position or fanning out money.
(Baumgarten and Strebel 2016)

1.2.3.6 Graphomotor Skills

For graphomotor skills, the functional interaction between the trunk muscles, the joints, and the muscles of the upper extremity is important. Combined and dosed dynamic push and pull movements enable the writing movement through co-contraction of all acting muscles.

The McMaster Handwriting Protocol distinguishes the following types of grips based on age (Pollock et al. 2008):

- radialpalmar grip (Fig. 1.23a)
- palmar supination grip (Fig. 1.23b)
- pencil grip with inwardly turned fingers
- brush grip
- pencil grip with extended fingers

- thumb grip (Fig. 1.23c)
- static tripod grip
- fourfinger grip
- lateral tripod grip
- dynamic tripod grip (Fig. 1.23d)

In graphomotor skills, the hand is divided into two halves:

- The radial side, which includes the thumb, index, and middle fingers.

They are important for the precision of the writing movement.

- The ulnar side, which includes the ring and little fingers.

They are responsible for the strength of the writing movement and for good guidance or stabilization of the hand.

1.2.3.6.1 Child Development of Graphomotor Skills

1.5 to 2 years
Toddlers develop an interest in the pencil. This is initially held in the **radial-palmar grip,** the **palmar supination grip** or **with inwardly**

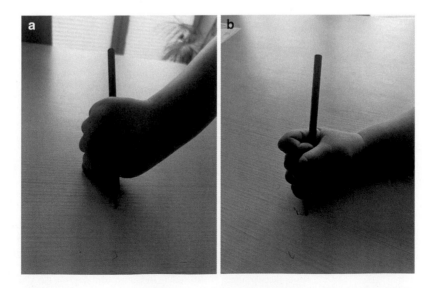

Fig. 1.23 **a** Radialpalmar grip, **b** palmar supination grip. (© Kinderkrankenhaus Wilhelmstift, with kind permission)

turned fingers (Fig. 1.23a,b). The drawing movements are undifferentiated and performed with inwardly rotated, pronated movements of the entire arm. Scribble pictures are created that go beyond the paper. Points and holes are produced with the pencil.

2nd year of life

In this phase of life, the toddler begins to vary the pencil grips into the **brush grip,** the **thumb grip** (Fig. 1.24), the **static three- or four-point grip** or into a **pencil grip with extended fingers.** In doing so, the toddler learns to guide the pencil from the elbow and the wrist. The lines rarely cross the sheet. First shapes like circles, zigzag lines or spirals are created. These are usually very rough and undifferentiated. Rotation, push, pull, and spiral movements are trained, which become more differentiated, coordinated, and finer in further development. They form the prerequisite for good letter formation and dynamic graphomotor skills.

3rd year of life

From the third year of life, the grip increasingly occurs in the **tripod grip.** In addition to the circles and spirals, isolated lines are added, which can be guided vertically or horizontally. The toddler begins to cross these lines and form squares or rectangles. This requires a good body schema and good visual perception. The lines and shapes are now combined into stick figures.

4th Year of Life

The child manages to hold the pencil appropriately in the precise **lateral** or **dynamic tripod grip** (Fig. 1.25). Shapes are colored in, footed heads are created. The drawing of objects begins. They are still wildly scattered on the sheet, but increasingly stay within the boundary. Spatial assignment does not yet take place. The child shows a solid hand dominance.

5th Year of Life

The drawn pictures enter into a spatial relationship. Objects are adequately arranged on the paper. Precise coloring is now possible. Interest

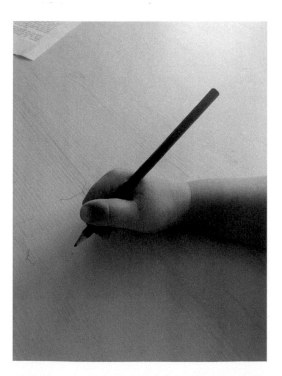

Fig. 1.24 Thumb grip. (© Kinderkrankenhaus Wilhelmstift, with kind permission)

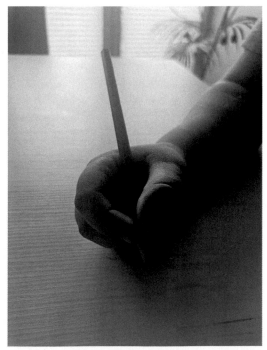

Fig. 1.25 dynamic tripod grip. (© Children's Hospital Wilhelmstift, with kind permission)

in letters begins. As a rule, children master the basic shapes by the age of five. This requires good force control, accuracy, fine motor coordination, and visuomotor skills. The drawing and writing movement is differentiated. A good interplay between the stability of the trunk and the mobility in the arm has developed. Lines are appropriately broken off and started to draw corners or circles in a differentiated way. For a dynamic handwriting, the continuous pattern must be well practiced. By the time of school enrollment, the child should have developed a holding hand and a functional hand. The paper must be held firmly with one hand so as not to slip during the writing process. Good hand-to-hand coordination is necessary for this, which the child has already practiced in the early stages of life (Pauli and Kisch 2012).

Malformations of muscles or joints, contractures, injuries, or neurological deficits impair the dynamic gripping patterns. Consultation with surgeons and therapists about possibilities for functional improvement is important. In the case of malformations, not only is mobility often restricted. Writing is additionally impaired by:

- lack of force control due to too much or too little force, often associated with pain,
- difficulties in dynamic and coordinated graphomotor skills,
- a changed or restricted development of hand dominance
- hyper- or hyposensitivity in the tactile and proprioceptive system,
- lack of eye-hand and hand-hand coordination,
- restricted targeted gripping,
- no crossing of the midline and thus restrictions in laterality,

1.3   Sensory Systems

The senses such as touch, taste, smell, balance, hearing, and sight develop intrauterinely in this order (Zimmer 2001). The sense of touch, taste, and smell develop from the second month of pregnancy. The sense of balance and hearing are added in the third month of pregnancy. The sense of sight develops from the fifth month of pregnancy. Postnatally, the infant is exposed to various stimuli that are filtered and processed. Thus, various motor functions and sensory impressions are interconnected and integrated in the development of the gripping function. Malformations can hinder this process. For a good gripping function, a mature finger identification is necessary. Children with a perception disorder often perceive the individual fingers as a whole and have difficulty moving the fingers selectively.

To better understand the influence of the sensory systems on the development of the gripping function, they are briefly explained.

A distinction is made between near and far senses:

The near senses include:

- the tactile-protopathic,
- the proprioceptive,
- the visceral,
- the vestibular system.

The far senses include:

- the tactile-epicritic,
- the olfactory,
- the gustatory,
- the auditory,
- the visual system.

▶ Even the unborn child feels, perceives, and reacts to perception (Schaefgen 2007).

1.3.1   Near Senses

1.3.1.1 Tactile-protopathic System

With surface sensitivity, we perceive skin stimuli such as heat, cold, vibration, pain, and touch. Not only is the reception of these stimuli taking place, but also their modulation. This creates a negative or a positive feeling. The object in the hand is sensed, experienced, and stored in its surface, texture, and consistency. For example, an infant perceives tactile stimuli on the hand when it supports itself in a prone position and feels the texture of the ground, when cuddling with a stuffed animal, or when reaching for a toy. A weakness in this system can lead to hypo- as well as hypersensitivity and thus impair a good gripping function. If a child is hypersensitive in tactile perception, it shows a defense and avoids these stimuli. In the case of hyposensitivity, the child deliberately seeks stimuli, but lacks the adequate dosage in dealing with objects and materials.

1.3.1.2 Proprioceptive System

Deep sensitivity is important for position sensation in combination with movement and force sensation. Through it, the extent of movement and force are controlled and coordinated. Good proprioception affects isolated finger movement with appropriate contraction and co-contraction. In addition, proprioception positively influences finger coordination, which allows targeted gripping and bilateral manipulation. The infant first learns to develop good postural control through gross motor movements. This includes lifting the head in the prone position and lifting the arms and legs from the ground. When the control of the trunk allows dynamic movement of the limbs, the infant can use the limbs for targeted, differentiated manipulation of toys. Pehoski describes the proximal-distal principle in this context (Pehoski 1992). If, for example, there is no appropriate postural control due to muscular changes, but a hypo- or hypertonus or restrictions in tonus regulation, the child has difficulties in achieving a dynamic fine and graphomotor function in the course of its development. In the case of hypotonia, the child tends to compensate for the low tension by cramping. In the case of hypertonia, the tense muscles do not allow dynamic fine motor use of the hand. A lack of proprioceptive perception of the movement of muscles, tendons, and joints leads to restrictions in force dosing. The children use too much force when they feel too little input, and too little force when they are hypersensitive to deep-sensitive input. An impairment in deep sensitivity results in children having difficulties

in target accuracy. Their actions are clumsy and uncoordinated.

1.3.1.3 Visceral System

The perception of the internal organs plays a role in well-being. Learning is limited in case of discomfort or unfulfilled needs. Malformations of the extremities often occur in combination with malformations of the internal organs.

1.3.1.4 Vestibular System

The vestibular system ensures good balance regulation. It provides feedback on the position or movement of the head in relation to gravity. The vestibular system has a major influence on oculomotor function and is therefore an important system for good eye-hand coordination and targeted gripping. For example, if a limb is not developed or if a prosthetic device is used, this affects the vestibular system.

1.3.2   Far Senses

1.3.2.1   Tactile-epicritical System

This system allows objects and surfaces to be touched, experienced, and distinguished. It is, for example, important for good stereognosis (the recognition of objects without visual control). If there is a disorder in this system, visual control can help, but sudden unexpected touches can be perceived as very unpleasant or even painful. Stereognosis is limited and surfaces or objects cannot be safely distinguished or feel unpleasant. Infants, toddlers, or children with hyper- or hyposensitivity in this area often avoid exploring new objects in their environment and avoid stimuli.

1.3.2.2 Olfactory System

Smelling is very important for the infant. It conveys security with familiar smells. This security motivates the infant to explore his environment. The cuddly toy has its own smell and is perceived and grabbed by the infant when it is nearby. The parents have a unique smell that is intensely perceived by the infant. The daily lunch smells and motivates to play with the spoon. Hyper- or hyposensitivity leads to avoidance of contacts with other people or reduces the desire for exploration (= the willingness to explore the environment).

1.3.2.3 Gustatory System

This system is closely related to the olfactory one. The gustatory system is, among other things, responsible for distinguishing between bitter, sweet, sour, and salty. The sense of taste stimulates playing with food or bringing food to the mouth.

1.3.2.4 Auditory System

Infants show a strong interest in sounds. They turn their head or the whole body in the direction from which the sound comes. This motivates to turn or crawl to get to the source of the sound. In addition, sounds stimulate interest in gamse when, for example, toys are repeatedly knocked against the floor or music sounds when buttons are pressed. Sounds are distinguished and the activity is constantly repeated. In this way, infants simultaneously train force dosing and various gripping forms.

1.3.2.5 Visual System

Visual perception is a prerequisite for targeted gripping. Good visual perception includes, for example, basic figure perception, form constancy, spatial position, spatial relationship, and spatial imagination. The infant learns to recognize the toy, target it, and grip it specifically. In the course, he also recognizes a certain toy in a pile of toys and can specifically reach for it. By the ninth month, infants can grasp features of objects and understand spatial relationships (Rosblad 2006). In the prone position, the infant learns to stabilize the head and simultaneously grip a targeted toy. These are the first steps for good eye-hand coordination. If the head or trunk cannot be adequately stabilized or if the limb is too short to bring the hand in front of the face or

to the mouth, this has a negative effect on eye-hand coordination. The following is an overview of the important developmental steps by months in relation to the gripping function.

1.3.3   Sensory Perception Processing Disorder (SPPD)

Children can show various abnormalities in perception processing, which can be assigned to the following examples according to their appearance and symptoms:

Sensory Regulation Disorder/Modulation Disorder

- Sensory Hypersensitivity/Stimulus Filter Disorder
- Sensory Hyposensitivity/Registration Disorder
- Sensory Stimulus Search

Sensomotor Disorder

- Postural Disorder/Postural Dyspraxia
- Coordination Disorder/Balance Regulation Disorder
- Motor Planning Disorder

Sensory Discrimination Dysfunction

- Visual Discrimination Disorder/Visual Perception Processing Disorder
- Auditory Discrimination Disorder/Auditory Perception Processing Disorder
- Tactile Discrimination Disorder/Tactile Perception Processing Disorder (Schaefgen 2012)

1.4   Developmental Phases by Months

Table 1.8 summarizes the developmental steps considered as the norm according to the literature. Deviations from the norm are the rule.

Table 1.8 Developmental phases by months

Month:	Trunk/Arms:	Hands:	Game Development/Sensory Systems:
1st month of life	The arms are usually flexed or extended at the elbow next to the body	• The hands are mostly loosely closed • Thumb adducted, sometimes loosely inclined (tucked in)	
2nd month of life	The arms are actively slightly raised in the supine position. This promotes the stability of the upper trunk	• Increased active opening of the hands • The infant cannot voluntarily let go of objects (hand-grasp reflex)	• The movements of the arms are perceived and the change in position is reported back to the brain • Experiencing the hands with the mouth serves to get to know one's own body. Therefore, hand-mouth contact is particularly important
3rd month of life	• Raising the arms in the supine position is possible, the hands are guided to the midline and visually fixed there. First phase of eye-hand coordination • Bringing the hands together trains the strength and endurance of the arms and the upper trunk. If a toy is also held in the hand, the infant needs more strength to lift the arms from the surface • Support on the forearms is possible, thereby strengthening the arms and upper trunk and promoting head control	• The hands are increasingly open and played with more • Individual touching of the thumbs and fingers with the mouth • Beginning selective movement of the fingers, first finger differentiation, infant feels that the hand is not a whole	• Toys are grabbed and played with aimlessly. This trains the infant in dynamic movement sequences and sensing changes in position • The infant realizes that he can achieve something with his activity • To promote hand-mouth coordination, the hands are touched with the mouth
4th month of life	• In prone position: more stable and symmetric	• Movements of the hands and fingers can occur independently of movements of the arm • Hands remain open when they lie next to the trunk in the supine position	• Through the prone position, the infant learns new position sensations, the vestibulum is stimulated • Uncoordinated grasping of offered toys as well as involuntary release • Play arches are touched and played with through uncoordinated unintentional movements • Increased visual fixation and tracking of toys promotes eye-hand coordination and targeted grasping • The infant looks at his toy and sees what happens with it • Alternation between visual observation and touching with the mouth • The hands touch each other when brought together in the center of the body, beginning hand-hand coordination. This trains arm control and endurance

(continued)

Table 1.8 (continued)

Month:	Trunk/Arms:	Hands:	Game Development/Sensory Systems:
5th month of life	• In the prone position, the baby becomes more secure in supporting itself on its forearms, controlling its head, and stabilizing its torso • Stabilization in an asymmetric support is now possible. This allows the baby to bring toys closer to itself with the other arm	• In the supine position, the hands are used to explore and perceive the body • The baby does not yet reach its feet at this stage of life • The hands are now fully open. The thumb is extended, but still slightly adducted. Toys are grasped with the whole hand in a palmar grip	• Active and targeted grasping of toys without explicit offer • The baby consciously and purposefully plays with toy arches • By actively playing with toys, new stimuli are experienced, such as sounds from tapping on the floor or wiping across the floor. The baby feels resistance and movement impulses. This in turn encourages experimenting with the toy and expanding the range of motion • Perception increasingly occurs through touching with the hands, through seeing and hearing.—a toy held with one hand can be passed to the other hand
6th month of life	• Turning from the supine position to the prone position and back is possible. This requires good motor planning, body coordination, and torso stability • In the prone position, the baby begins to rise from forearm support symmetrically into a broad-based wrist support. This strengthens the torso muscles • The body's center of gravity is further shifted towards the lower extremities. This requires good torso stability and strength in the arms, as well as stability in the wrists • Beginning to turn around its own axis and slide backwards • The range of motion of the arms is ever larger and stronger, objects are thrown out of reach	• In the supine position, the baby plays with its feet using its hands. This trains the abdominal and leg muscles • In the palmar grip, the baby manages to extend the thumb better and bring it into opposition • The thumb is still slightly adducted	• Alternating experience of objects with mouth, eyes, hands, and feet • Unpleasant surfaces are distinguished from pleasant ones
7th month of life	• The integration of flexion and extension patterns is complete • In the prone position, the weight in the broad-based wrist support is asymmetrically shifted to one side, so as to grasp with the other hand. The baby moves by rolling over the side	Continued grasping in the palmar grip, this is increasingly coordinated	• Toys are also grasped outside of reach • First understanding whether one or two objects are being held

(continued)

Table 1.8 (continued)

Month:	Trunk/Arms:	Hands:	Game Development/Sensory Systems:
8th month of life	The shoulder joints can be freely moved in all directions. Supination in the forearm is possible	• The grip develops from the undifferentiated palmar grip to the differentiated pincer grip • In the supine position, an object can be held in each hand	• Clapping, hiding, or picking up games are popular at this stage of development. They promote the coordination and perception of the hands, the targeted release, the dosage of force, the dynamics, rhythm, and interaction • The baby understands that a reaction follows its action
9th month of life	The baby begins to explore its surroundings by crawling. This promotes body coordination	In the supine position, the baby practices moving toys from the palm to the fingertips and passing objects from one hand to the other in a three-point or pincer grip	A holding hand and an action hand develop
10th month of life	• During this month of life, the infant manages to move from the prone position to the symmetrical quadruped position. In doing so, he supports himself in the mature hand support. The contact with the ground is further reduced, the erection against gravity succeeds. This leads to the development of asymmetric crawling and sitting. Later on, the infant manages to pull himself up symmetrically on furniture • Crawling is important for body coordination. Training of simultaneous tension and relaxation of interacting muscles (co-contraction). Good stability in the trunk and in the joints is important for this	• The handling and experimenting with movable objects, such as knobs, increases, practicing pro- and supination • The pincer grip becomes more coordinated and targeted, so that now even small things can be picked up • Practice of co-contraction (simultaneous relaxation and tension of interacting muscles), this is important for good fine coordination and a prerequisite for later use of a pen	• Infants at this age prefer to eat with their hands, mashing and smearing with porridge. This provides intense tactile stimuli and promotes fine motor skills • Independent drinking with both hands from a cup places high motor demands on the skill, the dosing of force, the planning of motor skills, the accuracy and the hand-mouth, as well as the hand-hand coordination
11th month of life	In standing, while supporting itself on furniture, asymmetric actions are performed, for example, by releasing one hand to grab a toy. This trains the trunk stability and the targeted, independently guided movement of an arm	Selective extension of the index finger and independent, selective movement of the fingers is possible. The fine coordination becomes more differentiated	Trying out cutlery, the infant begins to eat with a spoon. This trains the hand-mouth coordination
12th to 15th month of life	• Start of walking, this should be completed by the 18th month of life • Pushing and pulling of toys trains dynamic pressure and pulling movements with the arms against resistance • Better control over movements of the arms in rotation of the shoulder as well as pro- and supination in the forearm	• The thumb is in good opposition, small fluff, crumbs or stones are picked up from the ground in a pincer grip • Varying, practicing and differentiating various gripping techniques	• Plug cubes are intensively played with, which trains the eye-hand coordination. Manipulating the plug cubes practices fine coordination and the differentiated turning of objects in the hand • Independent eating with the spoon succeeds, the spoon is still held in pronation

(continued)

Table 1.8 (continued)

Month:	Trunk/Arms:	Hands:	Game Development/Sensory Systems:
15th to 18th month of life	A differentiated pro- and supination in the forearm is not yet possible and is always accompanied by a rotational movement in the shoulder	• The pincer grip becomes more secure, the fine coordination more differentiated • The toddler can turn thin pages of a book	• The toddler begins to show interest in pens (see graphomotor skills) • The training of eye-hand, hand-mouth, as well as hand-hand coordination has a positive influence on eating with a spoon, for example, the toddler manages to pick up food with the spoon and bring it to the mouth
18 months to 2 years of life	Movements from the elbow, forearm and wrist continue to be performed with the involvement of the shoulder. A selective movement from the elbow, forearm, wrist and fingers is only possible later	One hand is increasingly preferred. Pens are held in a fist grip or in the palmar grip in pronation of the forearm (see graphomotor skills)	• The development of the holding and action hand is becoming more evident • Beginning execution of bimanual activities as well as simultaneous handling of several small toys • Increased imitation of parents, for example in housework • Packing and unpacking games are popular • Independence increases. The removal of pants and socks succeeds
2nd to 2.5 years	Movements can be executed more independently from the elbow and wrist	The hand preference becomes clearer	• The confidence in hand-to-hand coordination increases. Interest in transferring games with water and sand, which promotes pro- and supination • Experimenting with scissors and fork • Two-handed work becomes more skillful, the toddler threads large beads onto a chain • Twist caps can be opened
3rd to 4th year		The hand preference is often mature by the end of the 3rd year of life and should be completed by the time of school enrollment	• Undressing is completely possible alone • Independent operation of simple buttons and zippers • The handling of scissors is safer
4th to 5th year		A working and holding hand is firmly integrated	• Coordinated and more differentiated finger movements. Small stones can be collected in one hand (see In-Hand Manipulation by Exner) • Threading of small beads is now successful. Learning to tie knots • Paper is torn with both hands, the handling of scissors is safer • Catching a ball is now possible without body use, only with the hands

(continued)

Table 1.8 (continued)

Month:	Trunk/Arms:	Hands:	Game Development/Sensory Systems:
5th to 6th year			• The interest in craft work increases • The child manages to cut out circles drawn on a paper along the line • Tying bows and brushing teeth can be done independently • The handling of cutlery becomes safer
6th to 7th year		Overall, the hand motor skills are now mature. The children can use their hands in a differentiated and skillful way	• By the time of school enrollment, the physiological use of the pen should be possible. (see Graphomotor Skills) • The use of the eraser is possible with measured force

Knowledge of the developmental steps allows conclusions to be drawn about the need for intervention.

1.5   Basics of Manual Therapy in Children

Unlike adults, children do not stay still during manual treatment. Therefore, many basic treatment aspects in adults cannot be transferred to children. Structure of manual therapy in adults:

Traction/ Compression
Push-Pull Technique/ Oscillation
Translatory Gliding
3 D Mobilisation

For adults, the following applies:

- If the moving joint partner is concave and the fixed joint partner is convex, osteokinematics (movement of bones in space) = arthrokinematics (movement of joint surfaces relative to each other) and a co-directional movement principle applies.
- If the moving joint partner is convex and the fixed joint partner is concave, osteokinematics ≠ arthrokinematics and an opposite movement principle applies.

In our adapted manual therapy for children, we also work with a fixed and a moving joint partner. However, the convex/concave rule is considered to a lesser extent. In infants and toddlers, our focus is more on stretching the structures (muscles, tendons, ligaments, and capsules) under gentle traction. This requires a firm grip and limits the scope for different manual techniques. Furthermore, it must be noted that the joints and soft tissues of the children described in this book do not conform to the norm and many manual techniques can only be applied in a modified form.

During the stretching, also in children a passive distinction can be made between the different end feelings of soft, springy, firm, and bony: If a bony end feeling is felt during passive stretching, the maximum permissible movement of the joint has been reached in an adult. From our experience, splinting and manual treatment in infants and toddlers is promising even when the bony end feeling is detected. The manual therapy and splinting should be maintained for at least one year to be able to measure success.

With a soft or springy passive end feeling, stretching of the structures in infants and toddlers is already promising through manual therapy alone and can be supported by splint treatment as needed.

The following applies:

If the passive range of motion is greater than the active one, the problem is more likely muscular.

If the passive and active range of motion are the same, the problem is more likely in the capsule, the ligaments, or the cartilage.

For children with normally developed joints, the older the children get, the more classical manual therapy can be included in the treatment. This applies not only to malformations but also to treatments after surgical interventions or injuries that result in restricted movement.

Convex	curved outward
Concave	curved inward
Osteokinematics	Movement of bones in space
Arthrokinematics	Movement of joint surfaces relative to each other
Traction	Pulling apart of a joint
Compression	Pressing together of a joint
Push-Pull Technique/ Oscillation	intermittent traction and compression impulses
Translatory Gliding	linearly guided sliding, the joint parts are moved parallel to each other
3 D Mobilisation	physiological initiation of movement from passive to assistive (supportive) to promote self-control

References

Baumgarten A, Strebel H (2016) Ergotherapie in der Pädiatrie. Schulz-Kirchner Verlag GmbH, Idstein

Bommas-Ebert U, Teubner P, Voß R (2011) Kurzlehrbuch Anatomie und Embryologie. Thieme, Stuttgart

Kapandji A (2016) Funktionelle Anatomie der Gelenke. Thieme, Stuttgart

Marzi I (2006) Kindertraumatologie. Steinkopff, Darmstadt

Neumann H (1963) Zur Verletzung des Fingerendgliedes und dessen biologischer Schienung durch die Nagelplastik. Mschr. Unfallheilk. 66

Oberg KC, Manske PR, Tonkin MA (2015) The OMT classification of congenital anomalies of the Hand and Upper Limb. Hand Surg 20(3):336–342

Pauli S, Kisch A (2012) Geschickte Hände Grund Skript. Verlag modernes lernen, Dortmund

Pehoski C (1992) Central nervous system control of precision movements of the hand. In: Case-Smith J, Pehoski C (Hrsg) Development of hand skills in the child (S 1–11). The American Occupational Therapie Association, Rockville

Pollock N, Lockhart J (2008) Mc-master handwriting protocol. McMaster University, Toronto

Pschyrembel 257 Auflage (1994) Hildebrandt, Helmut und Willibald, Berlin, New York: de Gruyter Verlag und Hamburg: Nikol Verlagsgesellschaft

Rosbald B (2006) Reaching and eye-handcoordination. In Henderson A, Pehoshki C (Hrsg) Handfunktion in the child. mosbyt, St Louis

Schaefgen R (2007) Praxis der sensorischen Integrationstherapie. Thieme, Stuttgart

Schaefgen R (2012) Skript Modul 1B der SI-Weiterbildung. Gesellschaft für Praxisbezogene Fortbildung, Bergen/Dumme

Schmidt HM, Lanz U (2003) Chirurgische Anatomie der Hand. Thieme, Stuttgart

Strassmair M, Wilhelm K, Hierner R (2009) Angeborene Fehlbildungen der Hand. Springer, Berlin

Tillmann BN (2020) Atlas der Anatomie des Menschen. Springer, Berlin

Waters PM, Bae DS (2012) Pediatric hand and upper limb surgery. Lippincott Williams & Wilki, Philadelphia

Wehr M, Weinmann M (2005) Die Hand/Werkzeug des Geistes. Elsevier GmbH

Zimmer K (2001) Das Leben vor dem Leben. Die körperliche und seelische Entwicklung im Mutterleib. Kösel, München

Zumasch R, Wagner M, Klausch S (2012) Anatomie und Biomechanik der Hand. Thieme, Stuttgart

Mail Literature

https://www.dimdi.de/dynamic/de/klassifikationen/icf/

Longitudinal Reduction Defect of the Radius

2

Contents

2.1 Clinical Picture

A radial longitudinal reduction defect (RLD), also known as clubhand, is a malposition of the wrist due to underdevelopment or absence of the radius (radial hypoplasia or aplasia) (Figs. 2.1 and 2.2). The forearm and hand are not or only partially developed on the radial side. This means that all radial structures, not just the bones, but also muscles, tendons, and nerves are affected. The carpus lacks support and the hand is in the so-called clubhand position, i.e., radial and palmar to the ulna. The ulna is curved in many cases. The forearm is significantly shortened. The soft tissues are highly altered. The radial wrist extensors have regressed to a tight, undifferentiated connective tissue structure. These shortened connective tissue strands and fasciae pull the hand into the malposition and the weak remaining hypoplastic extensors allow only a slight or no dorsal extension. The more pronounced the radius malformation, the more severe the soft tissue changes. The supination and pronation movement of the forearm is restricted or abolished in many cases. The fingers are also affected by the malformation: The thumb is usually hypoplastic or completely absent (exception TAR syndrome) (Fig. 2.2) and finger mobility is restricted in many cases, most strongly on the radial side and least on the ulnar side. The ring and little fingers are always the most mobile. The pinch grip is usually performed with the little and ring fingers.

The clinical classification divides the radial clubhand into four main types (Bayne and Klug 1987) (Fig. 2.2):

Type 1: slight distal radius shortening
Type 2: radius with severe shortening
Type 3: subtotal radius aplasia
Type 4: complete radius aplasia

The radial hypoplasia or aplasia can affect one or both arms. If it occurs in both arms, its severity can vary. The shoulder area, upper arms, and elbow joints can also be altered in very severe forms.

The clubhand can occur in isolation on one or both sides.

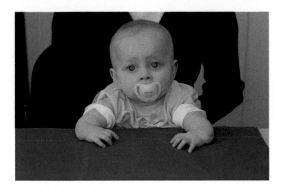

Fig. 2.1 9-month-old boy with bilateral radial longitudinal reduction defect (RLD): radius and thumb aplasia and finger flexion contractures. (© Children's Hospital Wilhelmstift, with kind permission)

It is often part of a syndrome, e.g. in:

- TAR syndrome = Thrombocytopenia-Absent-Radius Syndrome: lack of platelets, missing radii with existing thumbs (Fig. 2.3)
- Holt-Oram Syndrome: RLD and heart defects
- VATERL Association: See VACTERL Association without heart defects
- VACTERL Association: The combination of the following malformations,

V- Vertebral anomalies
A- Anal atresia
C- Cardial defects
T- Tracheo-esophageal fistula (connection between the airway and esophagus)
E- Esophageal atresia (closure of the esophagus)
R- Renal anomalies
L- Limb anomalies
- Fanconi Anemia: Changes in blood count due to regression of the bone marrow, skin pigmentation, RLD, dwarfism

2.2 Treatment

The treatment strategy for optimal care of the children and their parents includes:

- thorough clinical examinations,
- if necessary, human genetic examination,
- coordination of the hand surgical treatment concept with the treatment of other malformations,
- collaboration between hand surgeons, hand therapists, and orthopedic technicians,

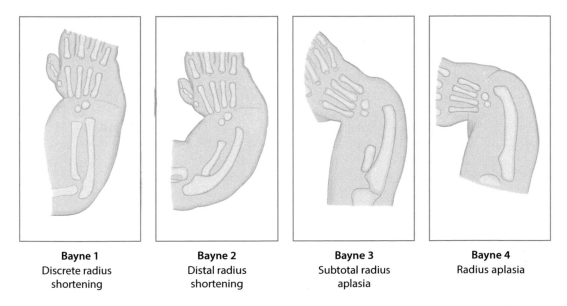

Bayne 1
Discrete radius shortening

Bayne 2
Distal radius shortening

Bayne 3
Subtotal radius aplasia

Bayne 4
Radius aplasia

Fig. 2.2 RLD classified based on the radiological development of the radius (Bayne, Klug). (From Hülsemann (expected 2023))

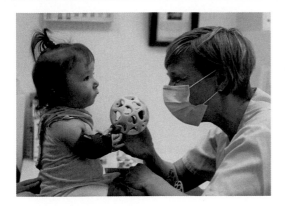

Fig. 2.3 9-month-old girl with bilateral RLD in TAR syndrome. On the right, the wrist is being stretched dorsally and laterally with a thermoplastic night splint. (© Children's Hospital Wilhelmstift, with kind permission)

- advice on self-help groups for information exchange between parents and growing patients.

The goals of treatment are:

- a straightening and, if possible, improvement of wrist mobility,
- a greater forearm-hand length,
- an improvement of the gripping function and the development of strength,
- the prevention of recurrences,
- satisfaction and independence of the child.

The goal is for both arms to be aligned with each other to better perform bimanual tasks in front of the body. With good arm length and straight hand position, food intake and body hygiene are much better possible, making the children more independent and less reliant on help.

The measures depend on the severity of the malformation, the possibilities of treatment, the age of the patient, and the wishes of the children and parents (Fig. 2.4).

A holistic functional analysis based on the **ICF** (Chap. 1) should not only be carried out at the beginning of treatment, but at regular intervals during growth. This can be used to check whether areas have changed and new goals need to be formulated.

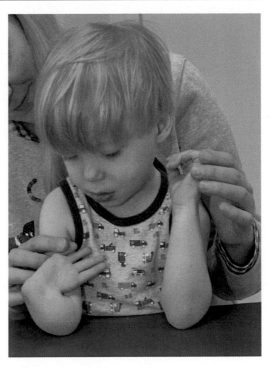

Fig. 2.4 3-year-old boy with RLD, severely shortened forearm, pronounced curvature of the ulna and thumb aplasia on the right. (© Children's Hospital Wilhelmstift, with kind permission)

▶ Early, continuous interdisciplinary support of parents and children is crucial for a permanently good result.

2.2.1 Treatment Concept

1. Already in the first year of life, the soft tissues at the wrist and possibly also the fingers are stretched by **splint treatments.** The passive and also active mobility of the elbow, hand and finger joints is improved by **manual therapy**.
2. Depending on the length of the forearm, the **surgical treatment** begins between the second and third year of life. In the first step, a **wrist distraction** using an external fixator pulls the wrist out of the malposition over several weeks and places it in front of the ulna. The increasing shortening of the flexor tendons is counteracted

by **manual stretching exercises** and in the case of stronger tendinogenic flexor contracture with a palmar **finger splint**. After achieving the desired position of the wrist, the fixator is removed and a **radialisation** (adjustment of the wrist on the ulna) is performed. A **Kirschner wire,** which extends from the metacarpus into the ulna, is inserted for temporary stabilization. A continuously worn **positioning splint** is made. It serves to secure the achieved erection and to protect the Kirschner wire. About 6 months after the radialisation, the stabilizing Kirschner wire is removed. If there is no thumb or if it is functionless, a **pollicization** is performed simultaneously in case of good active flexion ability of the ulnar fingers (Chap. 3). 5 weeks after the pollicization, intensive manual treatment and scar treatment of the new thumb begins. If the abduction of the thumb is insufficient, a **forearm splint** is made, which splints it in the desired position for another 12 to 16 weeks at night and stabilizes the wrist in the best possible passive/achieved erection. If no pollicization is performed, proceed with step 3.

3. To counteract the tendency of the wrist to reset during growth, **night positioning orthoses** are adapted in the best possible dorsal extension and ulnar deviation of the wrist and worn until growth is complete. Regular orthosis control is important to detect recurrences in time and to treat them if necessary.

4. Aids consultation (Chap. 7) is always useful during the growth and development of the child to promote independence.

▶ Examples depending on the developmental and therapy status illustrate the treatment steps—see end of the chapter.

2.2.2 Manual Therapy

Manual treatment primarily involves stretching the contractures of the elbow, wrist and finger joints. It is important to instruct the parents closely in manual stretching. They should perform the exercises several times a day.

The following should be noted in manual therapy:

- joint-near gripping of the joints to be stretched,
- daily performance of manual stretching, e.g. after each diaper change.

In addition to the wrist, depending on the movement restriction, the elbow and fingers 2–5 also need to be stretched in flexion and/or extension.

2.2.2.1 Manual Elbow Stretching

In the **manual stretching of the elbow**, the distal humerus is first palpated and grasped near the joint with one hand, and the distal ulna with the other hand. This is a prerequisite for good leverage (Fig. 2.5b). Now, depending on the restriction of movement in the elbow joint, a passive extension or flexion movement is performed (Fig. 2.5c):

- the proximal hand firmly grips the upper arm and holds it in a neutral position,
- the distal hand is the action hand and moves the child's forearm into the desired position.

At the end of the movement, depending on the severity of the contracture, a hard or soft springy stop is felt. At this point, the stretch should be slightly intensified and held.

> **Caution:**
> The mobility of the elbow is not only important for the child's independence, but also for the decision to surgically correct the wrist (Fig. 2.5a). Therefore, the treatment of the elbow has high priority.

2.2.2.2 Manual Wrist Stretching

In the **manual stretching of the wrist,** one hand palpates the distal ulna and the other hand palpates the proximal palm near the joint. Once the structures are firmly gripped, the wrist is stretched. For this:

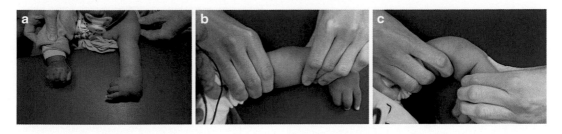

Fig. 2.5 **a** 17-month-old girl with RLD and left thumb aplasia in Noonan syndrome without active elbow mobility. **b** The humerus and ulna are palpated and grasped. **c** Stretching of the elbow into flexion. (© Kinderkrankenhaus Wilhelmstift, with kind permission)

- the hand on the child's forearm is the holding hand and
- the hand, which is at the level of the base joints, is the action hand.

The child's wrist is treated with:

- the action hand passively stretching it with slight traction to the dorsal and ulnar side. It is important that the hand firmly grips the palm, not the fingers, otherwise the base joints will be stretched too much to the ulnar side,
- the holding hand presses with the thumb on the ulnar head to achieve good leverage (Fig. 2.6a–c).

As soon as resistance is felt, the stretch is intensified, held for at least 10 to 20 seconds, and the movement is repeated as often as possible.

▶ In order to stretch tissue appropriately, the impulse on the structures must not be too weak. This stretch is held for about 10 to 20 seconds and repeated as often as possible.

Contracted tissue requires a lot of time to allow stretching, therefore splint treatment is needed at night for support.

2.2.2.3 Manual Stretching of Fingers 2 to 5

The focus of the **manual stretching of fingers 2 to 5** is on the joints that show a contracture. Mainly, the middle joints are affected by flexion contractures. The base joints tend to have extension contractures. The contracted joints are gripped close to the joint and stretched in the respective direction, depending on whether there is an extension or flexion deficit.

Stretching of the Middle Joints in Extension (Fig. 2.7)

- the therapist's proximal hand is the holding hand. It fixes the base joint,
- the therapist's distal hand is the action hand. It fixes the child's affected finger from the dorsal side with the index finger at the level

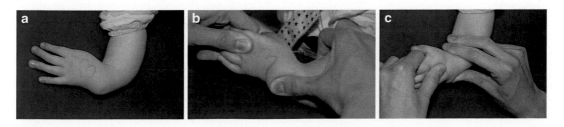

Fig. 2.6 **a** 3-year-old girl with bilateral RLD in TAR syndrome. **b** The distal ulna is palpated. **c** Stretching of the wrist to the ulnar and dorsal side. (© Kinderkrankenhaus Wilhelmstift, with kind permission)

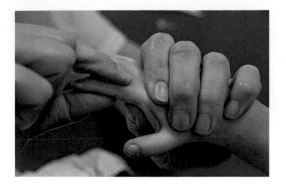

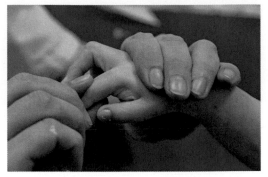

Fig. 2.7 Stretching of the middle joint into extension. (© Kinderkrankenhaus Wilhelmstift, with kind permission)

Fig. 2.8 Holding position for stretching the base joint into flexion. (© Kinderkrankenhaus Wilhelmstift, with kind permission)

of the head of the base bone and from the palmar side with the thumb at the level of the middle bone,
- the action hand stretches the middle joint to the maximum and then brings the base joint, if it is in a flexed position, into the neutral-zero position.

If a springy resistance is felt, the stretch is intensified and then held.

> **Caution:**
> The joints of the fingers should never be stretched into hyperextension, but always to the 0° position.
>   Particularly when stretching the middle joints, care should be taken that the base and end joints do not accidentally go into hyperextension.

Stretching of the Base Joints in Flexion (Fig. 2.8)

- the therapist's proximal hand (holding hand) fixes the head of the metacarpal bone of the affected finger in a sandwich grip, dorsally with the index finger and palmarly with the thumb,

- the therapist's distal hand (action hand) fixes the affected finger at the level of the distal base bone in a sandwich grip, that is, dorsally with the index finger and palmarly with the thumb,
- the action hand moves the child's affected finger with dorsal pressure on the base bone into the best possible flexion. If a springy resistance is felt, the stretch is intensified and then held.

▶ Every infant is different, so it is not always possible to stretch all structures at the given frequency with each diaper change.

2.2.3 Splint and Orthosis Treatment

2.2.3.1 Assessment of Wrist Mobility and Forearm-Hand Length

Night splints that keep the wrist in the best possible extension and upright position are used from about the 6th month of life to support manual therapy. As the children grow quickly, a constant adjustment of the splints must be made until the first surgical measure. Before manufacturing, the elbow mobility and the hand and forearm length are checked. The length of the forearm on the radial side is important. If the forearm is as long as the hand or longer, a

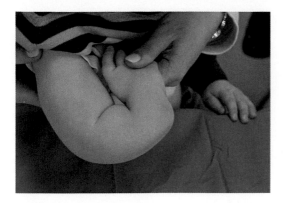

Fig. 2.9 2-year-old boy, RLD with severely shortened forearm, pronounced curvature of the ulna and thumb aplasia on the right/Assessment of elbow mobility and the length ratio of forearm and hand. (© Children's Hospital Wilhelmstift, with kind permission)

forearm palm splint is sufficient. If the forearm is shorter than the hand (Fig. 2.9), the upper arm must be included without restricting shoulder mobility. Subsequently, the maximum possible extension of the wrist is determined to the ulnar and dorsal side (Fig. 2.10a, b). A lot of force must be applied to stretch the firm structures as much as possible. Bony protrusions and prominent soft tissues must be detected by palpation to spare them in the splint.

> **Caution:**
> Forearm length radial side < hand length: the upper arm must be included in the splint to achieve sufficient leverage.

2.2.3.2 Holding Function for Adjusting an Upper Arm Palm Splint

For the manufacture of an upper arm splint, the holder encompasses the child's fingers with one hand, which are strongly pulled distally and ulnarly to align the wrist to the ulna. The child's fingers must lie next to each other and must not be crushed to prevent a flexion of the palm. With the other hand, the shoulder is encompassed and the entire arm is pulled into extension. With this longitudinal pull, the wrist is squeezed to the ulnar side and a rotation of the arm by the child is prevented (Fig. 2.11b). In addition, the holder indicates the upright position of the wrist to the dorsal side. He cannot achieve a maximum extension to the dorsal side, this must be done by the splint maker. A lot of force is required to stretch the wrist to the maximum (Fig. 2.11a).

2.2.3.3 Adjustment of an Upper Arm Palm Splint

The splint is now modeled around the arm on the radial side like a large clamp, while the longitudinal pull is maintained. The splint material is gently adapted to the soft tissues, only the palm is modeled with slight pressure to erect the wrist dorsally. As soon as the pre-stressed arm is released, it fits into the splint on the radial side, the "extension system" exists (Fig. 2.12b, c) (Chap. 8). By maintaining the radial extension tension of the arm in the splint, only a splint guide, i.e. the pressure from the radial side is needed and no further pressure point on the opposite ulnar side (Fig. 2.12b, c). The palmar pressure points are located on the palm and on

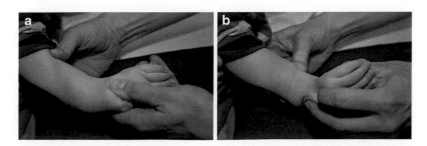

Fig. 2.10 **a** Extension of the wrist to the ulnar side, **b** Extension of the wrist to the dorsal side. (© Children's Hospital Wilhelmstift, with kind permission)

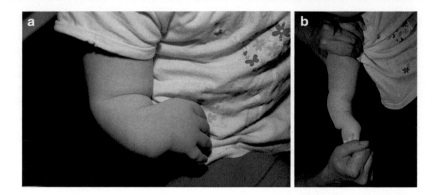

Fig. 2.11 a 18-month-old girl with RLD and thumb aplasia on the right, the forearm is shorter than the hand. **b** Grip technique for the production of a thermoplastic upper arm splint with a severely shortened forearm in RLD. (© Children's Hospital Wilhelmstift, with kind permission)

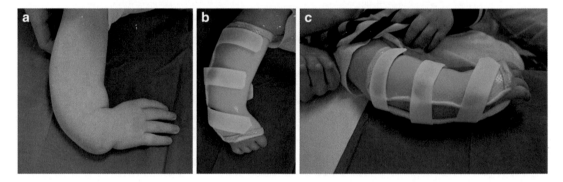

Fig. 2.12 a 2-year-old boy, RLD with a severely shortened forearm. **b** Same boy with a thermoplastic upper arm splint for stretching of the wrist. The arm is in extension tension in the splint. The splint encompasses his arm like a clamp. **c** No pressure point is needed on the ulnar side due to the radial extension tension. (© Children's Hospital Wilhelmstift, with kind permission)

the proximal forearm, the dorsal pressure point is located proximal to the wrist. A gentle fixation with Velcro straps holds the "clamp shape" together (Chap. 8). Padding at the level of the second metacarpal bone is necessary as the hand presses against the splint due to the resetting tendency (Fig. 2.12a). The fingers retain their free mobility.

> **Caution:**
> The splint material should only be lightly modeled due to the delicate, soft structures.

Upper Arm Palm Splint
- **Hand position of the holder:**
  Hand 1: Fingers 2–5 are pulled distally and ulnarly and lifted dorsally.
  Hand 2: The shoulder is gripped to prevent rotation, the elbow is extended.
- **Pressure points of the splint:**
  Radial = from the middle of the upper arm to the base joint of the index finger
  Ulnar = not necessary, as there is a longitudinal pull on the radial side (extension system in the clamp shape/Chap. 8)

Palmar = palm to proximal forearm
Dorsal = wrist to proximal forearm
- **Recommended materials** (Chap. 8)**:**
  – Thermoplastic material 2.0 mm (for
    very delicate arms 1.2 mm)
  – Velcro strap
  – Fleece strap
  – Possibly padding between the splint
    edges

2.2.3.4 Holding function for adjusting a forearm palm splint

If the forearm is as long as the hand or longer, a
forearm palm splint is sufficient (Fig. 2.13a, b).
To make the splint, the child's fingers are strongly
pulled distally and ulnarly and oriented dorsally,
so that the wrist is strongly ulnarly and slightly
dorsally erected. The child's fingers must not
overlap or be crushed, as this reduces the width
of the palm and the splint cannot optimally fit on
the palmar side (Fig. 2.13b). The upper arm and
the elbow are stabilized and a counterpressure on
the elbow is built up by the thumb of the holder.

This grip simultaneously prevents evasive movements by the child.

2.2.3.5 Adjustment of a Forearm Palm Splint

As with the upper arm palm splint, the clamp
shape has proven to be effective here (Chap. 8).
From the radial side, the material is modeled
around the hand and forearm, both palmar and
dorsal, leaving the ulnar side free. The pressure
points are located on the palmar side at the palm
and the proximal forearm, dorsally proximal to
the wrist and radially along the entire length,
proximal to the base joint of the index finger to
distal to the elbow (Fig. 2.14a). To achieve sufficient leverage, the splint must encompass the
forearm as much as possible without restricting
the movement of the elbow. An existing thumb
is generously spared. If it is hypoplastic, the
edges of the splint are padded, as pressure points
quickly develop on the unstable, very soft structures (Fig. 2.14b). Padding in the area of the
first interdigital fold or at the level of the second
metacarpal bone is necessary, as the hand in its
original position pushes radially and palmarly
into the malposition (Fig. 2.14a, b). The splint

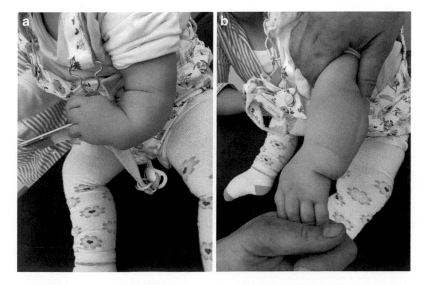

Fig. 2.13 a 11-month-old girl with RLD and thumb hypoplasia on the left. **b** Gripping function for the production of
a thermoplastic forearm splint in RLD. (© Children's Hospital Wilhelmstift, with kind permission)

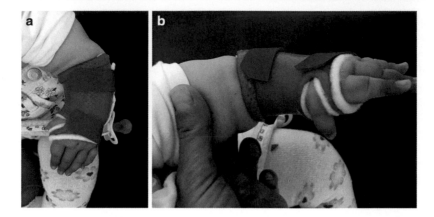

Fig. 2.14 **a** Thermoplastic forearm splint for expansion of the wrist in RLD. **b** Generous sparing of the hypoplastic thumb and padding of the first interdigital fold. (© Children's Hospital Wilhelmstift, with kind permission)

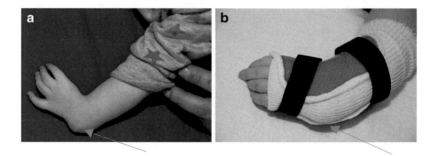

Fig. 2.15 **a** 23-month-old girl with RLD and thumb aplasia, with pronounced soft tissues on the ulnar head. **b** Same girl, thermoplastic forearm splint with sparing of the prominent soft tissues at the level of the ulnar head. The rein guide around the soft tissues ensures good fixation of the splint. (© Children's Hospital Wilhelmstift, with kind permission)

ends proximal to the base joints of the fingers, so as not to restrict their freedom of movement.

In many cases, the soft tissues at the level of the ulna head are prominent (Fig. 2.15a). Since even slight pressure on the ulnar head causes pressure points and shifts the soft tissues, the "clamp shape" through the "extension system" is the solution to this problem. The splint completely spares the ulnar head with the prominent soft tissues (Fig. 2.15b). In addition, a rein guide around the soft tissues can prevent the splint from slipping, especially if no thumb is present. Even during splint treatment, the desired extension of the radial soft tissues can lead to a

shortening of the flexors. The flexion contractures are specifically treated with manual therapy.

Forearm Palm Splint
- **Hand position of the holder:**
  Hand 1: Fingers 2-5 are pulled distally and ulnarly.
  Hand 2: fixes the upper arm with thumb pressure at the elbow, elbow is extended.
- **Pressure points of the splint:**
  Radial = from the proximal forearm to the base joint of the index finger

Ulnar = not necessary, as there is a longitudinal pull on the radial side (extension system in the clamp shape/ Chap. 8)
Palmar = from the palm to the proximal forearm
Dorsal = distal forearm
- **Recommended materials:**
  see Upper Arm Palm Splint

2.2.3.6 Forearm Orthosis with Finger Enclosure

If the fingers show strong flexion contractures in the middle joints, it is recommended to treat these with forearm orthoses with finger encasement (Fig. 2.16a, b). In addition to straightening the wrist, the varying degrees of flexion contractures of each individual finger must be precisely counteracted. Due to rapid growth, the first fitting is recommended after the first year of life. Prior to this, therapy is carried out using thermoplastic splints to stretch the wrist and manual therapy of all affected joints. Due to the complexity, these orthoses are made by orthopedic technicians from plaster casts (manufacture from plaster cast see Chap. 8). The orthosis has the task:

- to straighten the wrist as much as possible to the ulnar and dorsal side
- to hold the fingers
  - in the base joints at 0°,
  - in the middle joints in the best possible extension,
  - in the end joints in a suggested flexion of 10°,
  - and to spare an existing thumb.

The orthosis encompasses the hand and ends, depending on the length of the forearm, on the forearm or upper arm. Here too, the clamp shape has proven its worth (Chap. 8).

To prevent the hand from slipping away, the radial side is completely encompassed. This large pressure point prevents pressure sores. The fingers are individually encased. Differently pronounced finger contractures are compensated from the palmar side. The webs prevent skin-to-skin contact and the fingers from sliding radially (Fig. 2.16a, b). From the palmar side, each finger is straightened as much as possible and encased so that all base joints are at the same level. The common dorsal finger pad, which pushes the fingers between the base and middle joints into the orthosis, compensates for minor differences. The thumb is spared.

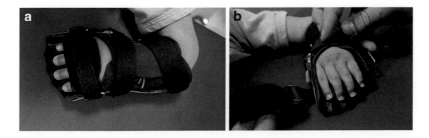

Fig. 2.16 a 18-month-old boy, with RLD and right thumb hypoplasia, forearm orthosis with individual finger encasement made of Streifi-Flex with carbon brace. The orthosis encompasses the wrist and the forearm as a semi-shell around the radial side, dorsally the forearm is held in the splint by the wide strap. From the dorsal side, the pad pushes the fingers into the orthosis at the level of the base joints, the elbow has free mobility. To fully utilize the forearm length and thus the lever, the orthosis is beveled on the proximal forearm—radially it is shorter than ulnarly. **b** The fingers are individually encased to counteract the different flexion contractures, the pad has guides for each individual finger. (© Children's Hospital Wilhelmstift, with kind permission)

Forearm orthosis with finger encasement

- **Hand and finger position in the orthosis:**
  Wrist—Extension to the dorsal (up to a maximum of 30° extension) and to the ulnar side.
  Fingers 2–5—Extension of the fingers in the base, middle and end joint up to a maximum of 0° with individual finger encasement, thumbs are generously spared.
- **Orthosis encasement:**
  Approximately 2/3 of the circumference of the forearm and hand are encased from the palmar side, proximally the orthosis is as long as possible radially and ulnarly without restricting movements, therefore usually a few centimeters longer on the ulnar side.
- **Pressure points:**
  Palmar: from the forearm to the fingertip. Differences in finger flexion contractures are compensated on the palmar side via the orthosis
  Dorsal: Closure at the level of the distal forearm close to the wrist, attachment on the proximal forearm, finger pad between base and middle joints
  Radially: proximal forearm to the fingertip of the index finger
  Ulnarly: distal forearm
- **Recommended materials** (Chap. 8):
  – Streifi-Flex
  – Carbon brace
  – Deflector
  – Strap with Velcro fastener
  – Finger pad

Caution:
Avoid deviation and hyperextension in the metacarpophalangeal joints. Different finger flexion contractures must be compensated for in the orthosis on the palmar side.

2.2.4 Functional improvement in severe forms of RLD

In the case of complete loss of elbow mobility, a non-existent elbow joint, or extremely short upper and lower arm, no functional improvement of the wrist can be achieved surgically (Fig. 2.17a, b). Improvement is possible with splints and manual therapy (Fig. 2.3). Aids support everyday life. In this severe form of RLD, the elasticity and mobility of fingers, wrist, elbow, and shoulder joint can be improved through constant therapy to achieve a larger range of motion. Whether surgical straightening of the hand is sensible must be carefully considered in these cases and reassessed repeatedly during growth. The clubhand position allows these children to eat and drink independently without outside help. Surgical straightening of the wrist would take away this important function. A functional analysis by occupational or physical therapists can be helpful for the decision to operate.

Caution:
In severe forms of malformation, surgical correction of the wrist can bring disadvantages for the child.

2.2.5 Surgical therapy and accompanying conservative treatment

2.2.5.1 Wrist Distraction

If surgery is indicated, depending on the child's growth, the wrist is straightened from the 2nd to 3rd year of life through radialization, centralization, or free toe joint transfer. As a preparation, wrist distraction is performed using a half-ring fixator (Fig. 2.18). The wrist is distracted onto the ulnar end over a period of 3 to 4 months, the radial soft tissues are thereby lengthened by 4 to 6 cm (Figs. 2.19a, b and 2.20a–c). With an initial length of the forearm of approx. 9

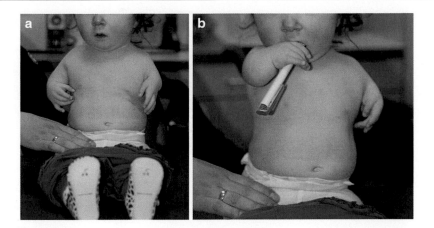

Fig. 2.17 a 9-month-old girl with bilateral RLD in TAR syndrome, extremely short arms and slender shoulder area. **b** The girl can bring her hand to her mouth due to the clubhand position. (© Children's Hospital Wilhelmstift, with kind permission)

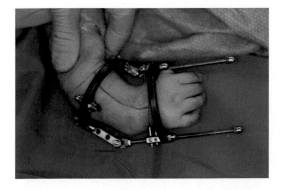

Fig. 2.18 3-year-old boy, intraoperatively, attachment of a half-ring fixator for wrist distraction. (© Children's Hospital Wilhelmstift, with kind permission)

cm, this means a significant increase in length and a strong stretching, especially of the flexor tendons. The individual surgical steps are effectively facilitated by the preceding splint treatment and manual therapy.

The goal of wrist distraction:

- Stretching of the radial soft tissues,
- thereby facilitating the surgical positioning of the carpus in front of the ulnar end,
- Relief of pressure on the distal ulnar growth plate.

This results in a greater forearm length.

During wrist distraction, the impending flexion contracture of the fingers must be counteracted and a deterioration of finger mobility prevented (Fig. 2.21a, b). This is achieved by stretching the fingers several times a day. If the stretching is too painful or the flexion contracture cannot be prevented by manual stretching, a palmar forearm-finger splint helps to counteract this. In addition, hand therapy is intensified and distraction is paused.

2.2.5.2 Manual Stretching of Fingers 2 to 5 During Wrist Distraction

During distraction with a length increase of 4 to 6 cm, the flexors often do not stretch sufficiently. They pull the fingers into flexion (Fig. 2.21a, b). Regular manual stretching of fingers 2–5 counteracts this. For stretching, the forearm is held by the fixator and the fingers are individually stretched (Fig. 2.22b, c). For this, the therapist's thumb pad supports the middle phalanx from the palmar side. The index finger is placed dorsally proximal to the middle joint and the middle joint is extended in this position with pressure (Fig. 2.22c). If the base joint is in flexion, it is slowly brought to the 0° position and thus the finger is maximally stretched. The

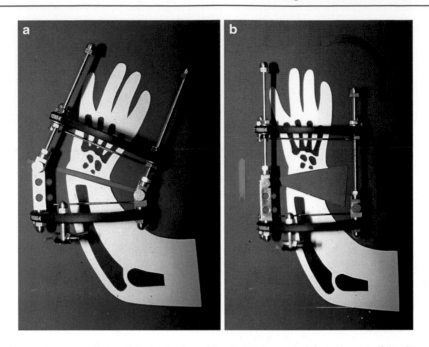

Fig. 2.19 a Schematic representation at the beginning of the distraction period. **b** At the end of the distraction period. The red arrows show the extent of the lengthening distally and ulnarly. (© Children's Hospital Wilhelmstift, with kind permission)

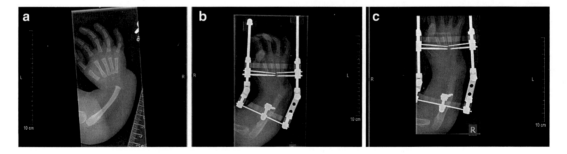

Fig. 2.20 a–c Clubhand in TAR syndrome: **a** At the age of 8 months, **b** at the beginning of distraction at the age of 23 months, **c** after 7 weeks of distraction. (© Children's Hospital Wilhelmstift, with kind permission)

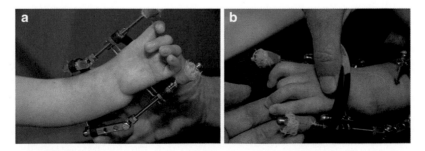

Fig. 2.21 a Finger flexion contractures during wrist distraction, palmar view, **b** dorsal view. (© Children's Hospital Wilhelmstift, with kind permission)

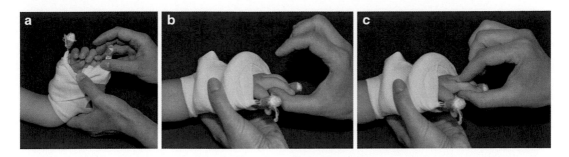

Fig. 2.22 a Bandaged half-ring fixator, flexion contractures of fingers 2–5. A self-adhesive bandage has been wrapped over the cap nuts for protection. **b** The forearm is fixed by the fixator, the middle joint is supported by the therapist's thumb pad from the palmar side. **c** The middle joint is brought into maximum extension by the counter-pressure of the index finger pad. (© Children's Hospital Wilhelmstift, with kind permission)

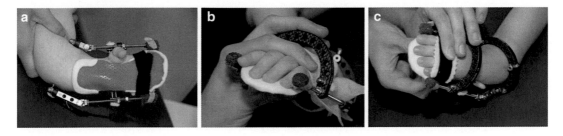

Fig. 2.23 a–c Palmar thermoplastic night resting splint for stretching fingers 2–5 during wrist distraction. Due to the straight shape at the proximal end, the splint can be pushed under the bandage. A strap on the base of the fingers is sufficient as the only attachment. (© Children's Hospital Wilhelmstift, with kind permission)

stretch should be held for 10 to 20 seconds and performed with each finger. Repetitions are done several times a day. Toddlers have no difficulty using the affected hand, even with a fixator, as a holding or functional hand (Fig. 2.22a). Objects are grasped between the fingers. If the affected hand is not used in everyday life, therapeutic intervention should be considered.

2.2.5.3 Finger Splint During Wrist Distraction

If daily manual stretching is not sufficient to prevent flexion contractures, a forearm-finger splint is made. It splints the fingers from the palmar side and ends on the proximal forearm. The shape of the splint is kept as neutral as possible at the forearm and wrist, as the position and shape of the wrist change during the course of distraction (Fig. 2.23a). This means that the splint contours are not modeled there,

but a contact surface is formed that is as straight as possible. Since the splint is pushed under the bandage, which fits tightly on the palmar forearm, a closure at the fingers is sufficient for a good fit (Fig. 2.23c). The dorsal closure presses the fingers between the base and middle joints into the splint (Fig. 2.23b, c). The fleece strap, which fixes the fingers in the splint, should also be well padded (Chap. 8), as pressure points can quickly develop from the strap. If there are different degrees of contractures on the individual fingers, these must be compensated for over the splint and not over the closure.

2.2.5.4 Splint Adjustment with Existing Half Ring Fixator

It makes sense to stretch the fingers before making the splint in order to achieve good extension of the fingers in the splint and to reduce pain during the making. The modeling of the splint

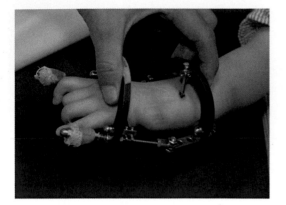

Fig. 2.24 The hand is fixed by gripping the fixator rings. This process is painless. (© Children's Hospital Wilhelmstift, with kind permission)

the fixator presses the splint to the forearm and thus fixes the proximal part of the splint.

- **Pressure points of the splint:**
  Palmar = finger to proximal forearm
  Dorsal = a soft pad presses the fingers between the base and middle joints into the splint
- **Recommended materials** (Chap. 8):
  - Thermoplastic material 2.0 mm
  - Velcro strap
  - (Elastic) Fleece strap
  - Edge padding
  - Padding under the fleece strap

is usually painful for the children, as tension is applied to the contracted tendons. Therefore, good fixation of the hand is all the more important. The holder fixes the arm by the fixator (Fig. 2.24) while the splint is quickly modeled. After a wearing time of 5 to 10 minutes, the newly made splint should no longer bother the child. If this is not the case, the splint must be made with less extension. The splint is worn during sleep, the rest of the day the fingers remain free. Since the wrist distraction changes the hand and finger position, it may be necessary to adjust the thermoplastic splint in the course of treatment. According to our experience, this is necessary a maximum of one to two times during the distraction time.

Finger splint during wrist distraction
- **Hand position of the holder:**
  Hand 1: Fixator is fixed by the half rings.
  Hand 2: Fixes the upper arm to prevent an evasive movement.
- **Splint coverage:**
  The splint is only made palmar from the fingertips to the proximal forearm. It is **not** modeled laterally around the hand or forearm. The bandage around

This type of splint can be applied and removed without changing the bandage by sliding it between the bandage and forearm or pulling it out. This facilitates daily handling.

2.2.5.5 Radialisation and K-Wire Fixation

After the distraction is completed, the external fixator is removed and a radialisation is performed. The carpal bones, which are located in front of the ulna due to the distraction (Fig. 2.25a), are fixed in this new position. The rudimentary radial wrist extensors are transposed to the ulnar carpus. The wrist is secured in this position by an intramedullary Kirschner wire (K-wire), which is inserted through the 2nd metacarpal bone and the carpus into the ulna (Figs. 2.25b and 2.26c). This Kirschner wire remains for about 6 months.

Postoperatively, a palmar forearm splint made of plaster is first applied. Due to the strong postoperative swelling, it is advisable to make a thermoplastic splint only 4 to 6 weeks postoperatively. Both the plaster splint and the thermoplastic splint must be worn day and night to keep the wrist in the new position and to protect the Kirschner wire. They may be removed during bathing and quiet activities under supervision, e.g. during eating.

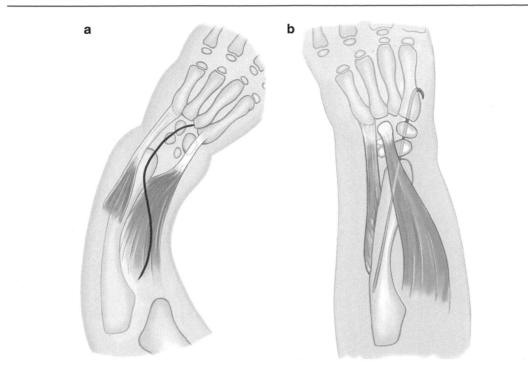

Fig. 2.25 a Schematic representation before radialisation. **b** Schematic representation after radialisation, fixation of the wrist with a K-wire. (© Children's Hospital Wilhelmstift, with kind permission)

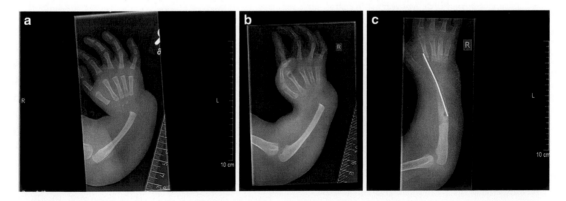

Fig. 2.26 a–c Clubhand in TAR syndrome **a** At the age of 8 months, **b** shortly before the start of distraction at the age of 22 months, **c** after removal of the fixator and after radialisation at the age of 25 months. The pin sites in the bone are still visible. (© Children's Hospital Wilhelmstift, with kind permission)

2.2.5.6 Forearm-Palm Splint during K-Wire Fixation

The splint to protect the Kirschner wire and the new wrist position is adjusted from the palmar side and covers at least 2/3 of the forearm circumference (Fig. 2.27a, b). Before making the splint, it must be checked whether the Kirschner wire can be felt under the skin at the 2nd metacarpal bone. If this is the case, a pad is stuck on the spot for the duration of the splint production. This creates the necessary cavity in the splint to prevent pressure points and/or skin irritations. Since the Kirschner wire determines the position of the wrist, the thermoplastic material may only

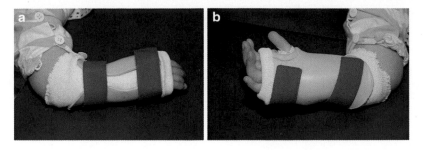

Fig. 2.27 **a** Thermoplastic forearm splint for fixation of the wrist after radialization and K-wire fixation from the dorsal and **b** palmar side. (© Children's Hospital Wilhelmstift, with kind permission)

be modeled around the hand without previously applying tension or pressure to the wrist. A splint thickness of 3.2 mm is recommended, as the children will play and romp with this splint for several months. The splint must withstand this strain.

Forearm-Palm Splint during K-Wire Fixation
- **Hand position of the holder:**
  Hand 1: Fingers 2–5 are held.
  Hand 2: Fingers fix the upper arm, it is only held so strongly that the splint maker can work at ease. No pull towards the dorsal or ulnar side, as the position is determined by the K-wire.
- **Splint coverage:**
  Approx. 2/3 of the circumference of the forearm and hand are covered. Proximally, the splint is as long as possible on the radial and ulnar sides, without restricting movements in the elbow. Therefore, usually it is a few centimeters longer on the ulnar side to achieve a maximum lever. The fingers remain free.
- **Pressure points of the splint:**
  Palmar side: from the forearm to the palm
  Dorsal side: around the wrist. The splint covers about half of the back of

the hand and the forearm on the dorsal side
Radial side: proximal forearm to proximal of the index finger base joint
Ulnar side: distal forearm
- **Recommended materials:**
  – Thermoplastic material 3.2 mm
  – Further materials: see Upper Arm-Palm Splint

2.2.5.7 Forearm Orthosis with Removable Finger Attachment

If the fingers are in a pronounced flexion position due to strong tendon tension, at the time of K-wire fixation an orthosis can be made that also splints the fingers. In order that the child can use the fingers during K-wire fixation, the finger attachment should be removable (Fig. 2.28c, d) and only be attached at night (Fig. 2.28a, b). A so-called "nose" (Chap. 8) on the ulnar side of the splint extends the hand rest during the day and thus prevents pressure points (Fig. 2.28c, d). It is designed in such a way that flexion is possible in all index finger joints. Pronounced tendon tension leads to an inclination of the wrist to the radial side despite the radialization and the K-wire fixation, hence the extended support is beneficial.

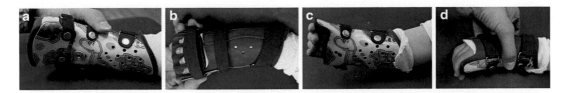

Fig. 2.28 **a–d** Forearm orthosis with removable finger attachment. The finger part is inserted into the forearm splint and fixed with a knurled screw. This allows the fingers to be stretched overnight. During the day, the finger attachment is removed to allow finger movements. The "nose" on the splint extends the pressure support of the hand on the radial side without restricting the movement of the fingers. (© Children's Hospital Wilhelmstift, with kind permission)

Forearm Orthosis with Removable Finger Attachment
- **Hand and finger position in the orthosis:**
  Wrist—as dictated by the K-wire, usually in a 0° position
  Fingers 2–5—Extension of the fingers in the base, middle, and end joint up to a maximum of 0° with individual finger inclusion, thumb generously spared
- **Orthosis length:**
  Approx. 2/3 of the circumference of the forearm and hand are enclosed from the palmar side, proximally the orthosis is as long as possible on the radial and ulnar side without restricting movements, therefore usually a few centimeters longer on the ulnar side.
- **Pressure points:**
  Palmar side with finger attachment: from the forearm to the fingertip. Differences in finger flexion contractures are compensated on the palmar side via the orthosis
  Palmar side without finger attachment: from the forearm to proximal of the finger base joints
  Dorsal side: Closure at the level of the distal forearm close to the wrist, attachment on the proximal forearm, finger pad between base and middle joints
  Radial side with finger attachment: proximal forearm to the fingertip of the index finger

Radial side without finger attachment: proximal forearm to approx. the middle joint of the index finger
Ulnar side: distal forearm
- **Recommended materials** (Chap. 8):
  - Streifi-Flex
  - Carbon brace
  - Deflector
  - Strap with Velcro fastener
  - Finger pad
  - Knurled screw

Caution:
Avoid deviation and hyperextension in the finger base joints. Different finger flexion contractures must be compensated in the orthosis via the palmar side.

2.2.5.8 Removal of the K-Wire and Pollicization

After approximately 6 months, the wire is removed. If no thumb is present or if it is severely underdeveloped (Fig. 2.29a), pollicization can be performed if the existing fingers have good mobility. In this process, the index finger is moved to the thumb position (Fig. 2.29b) (Chap. 3). Pollicization is a complex procedure. It takes about 5 weeks for the postoperative swelling to decrease. After this time, a thermoplastic night splint must be fitted to prevent a recurrence of the clubhand and to

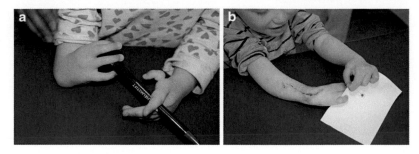

Fig. 2.29 **a** 3-year-old girl with RLD on both sides, thumb aplasia on the right and severe thumb hypoplasia on the left. The child grasps in a lateral grip (Chap. 1). **b** The same girl at the age of 5, after pollicization on the left and wrist distraction and radialization on the right. (© Children's Hospital Wilhelmstift, with kind permission)

support the pollicized thumb in the best possible abduction and opposition position. This splint is worn at night until the child has outgrown the splint, but at least for three months. In the first three to four months postoperatively, strong scar tension can pull the thumb into adduction. This must be counteracted by manual therapy, scar treatment, and splint therapy (Chap. 3).

2.2.6 Postoperative Treatment

2.2.6.1 Forearm Splint after Pollicization

The thermoplastic night splint, which is made after radialization and pollicization, extends from the forearm to the base joints of fingers 3 to 5. The mobility of the elbow must not be impaired. The splint is modeled from the dorsal side around the palm, the thumb, and the forearm. This technique leads the thumb into abduction and opposition (Chap. 3).

The middle finger and the thumb are in the best possible abduction and opposition to each other (as when gripping a bottle). The tip of the thumb should, if possible, face the ring finger to allow the best possible opposition to all fingers (Chap. 3). The wrist is in the best possible extension (0 – max. 30° dorsal extension) and can be slightly aligned to the ulnar side (10-20°) to counteract a wrist tilt to the radial side (Fig. 2.30a, b). This night splint should be worn from the 5th postoperative week for at least 3 months to counteract scar traction and achieve maximum abduction and opposition of the "new" thumb. When the child has outgrown the splint and the thumb is well positioned, splint treatment is continued to maintain wrist alignment – step 5. During the day, the hand is left free to allow the thumb to be used and to learn new gripping patterns (Fig. 2.31). This is promoted by hand therapy.

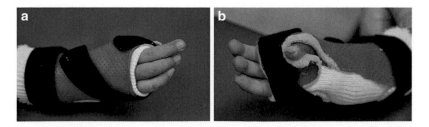

Fig. 2.30 **a** Thermoplastic splint for stabilizing the wrist and thumb after radialization and pollicization from the dorsal side and **b** from the palmar side, the tip of the thumb faces the pad of the ring finger. (© Children's Hospital Wilhelmstift, with kind permission)

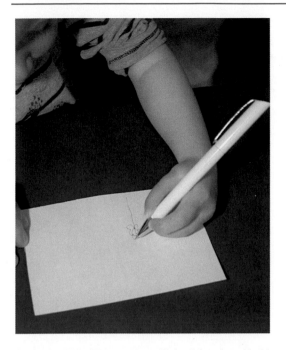

Fig. 2.31 The child uses the pollicized thumb and holds the pencil in the dynamic three-point grip (Chap. 1). (© Children's Hospital Wilhelmstift, with kind permission)

Forearm Splint after Pollicization

- **Hand and finger position in the splint:**
  Wrist – dorsal extension (up to a maximum of 30° extension) and ulnar deviation (up to a maximum of 20° ulnar deviation).
  Middle finger and "new" thumb – best possible abduction and opposition to each other.
- **Splint coverage:**
  Approximately 2/3 of the circumference of the forearm and hand are covered.
  Proximally, the splint is as long as possible on the radial and ulnar sides without restricting elbow mobility. Therefore, it is usually a few centimeters longer on the ulnar side to achieve a maximum lever.

"New" thumb: in the best possible abduction and opposition to the middle finger.

- **Pressure points:**
  Palmar side: palm and proximal forearm
  Dorsal side: firm pad at the proximal wrist, attachment on the proximal forearm
  Radial side: Proximal forearm up to the level of the base joint of the middle finger
  Ulnar side: proximal forearm and edge of the hand
  Thumb:
  – palmar side – base joint,
  – ulnar side – first phalanx,
  – radial side – first phalanx
  – dorsal side – first phalanx possibly up to the distal end joint, to slightly grasp it in flexion
- **Recommended materials:**
  see upper arm palmd splint

Caution:
Prevent hyperextension in the base joints of the middle finger and the "new" thumb

---

2.2.6.2 Forearm Orthosis Against Retraction Tendency

If no pollicization was performed, treatment with a night orthoses begins immediately after removal of the Kirschner wire. After a pollicization, this treatment begins about 3 to 6 months later. To counteract the tendency of the wrist to retract, the night orthoses must be worn until the end of growth. Depending on age and growth spurt, the child or adolescent needs new orthoses every few months to years. In kindergarten and primary school age, children shoot up in height and lose their "baby fat". Then it is possible that the orthoses are wide enough for a long time, but the length is no longer sufficient at some point. For a sufficient lever that keeps the wrist

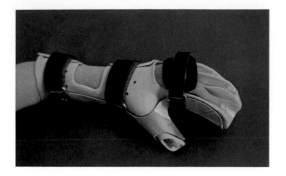

Fig. 2.32 Streif-Flex orthosis with carbon brace, to prevent the retraction tendency of the wrist, improve the flexion contractures of fingers 3–5 and secure the pollicized thumb in abduction and opposition. (© Children's Hospital Wilhelmstift, with kind permission)

in extension, the orthosis must have a length up to the proximal forearm. Therefore, it is advisable to offer an orthosis check at least once a year until the end of primary school age. During the plaster casting of the hand, the wrist must be brought into the best possible dorsal and ulnar alignment. This requires considerable force from the holder. Here, it is not advisable to work too timidly, otherwise a recurrence is favored.

In many cases, the children need a forearm orthosis with a palm enclosure for the night, which can be designed with a finger enclosure depending on the flexion contracture of the fingers. A thumb enclosure is advisable in the first postoperative year after pollicization (Fig. 2.32).

Forearm Orthosis Against Retraction Tendency

- **Hand position in the orthosis:**
  Maximum extension of the wrist to the dorsal (0–30°) and ulnar side (can be aligned into a slight ulnar deviation).
- **Orthosis coverage:**
  Approx. 2/3 of the arm circumference is enclosed.
  On the radial and ulnar side, the orthosis is as long as possible without restricting elbow mobility. Therefore, it is usually a few centimeters longer on

the ulnar side to achieve a maximum lever.
  Wrist = maximum extension towards the ulnar and dorsal side, the dorsal pad at the proximal wrist pushes the arm into the orthosis.
  Fingers (if necessary) = individual finger enclosure, contractures are compensated on the palmar side, dorsal pressure pad between the base and middle joints.
  Thumb (if necessary) = in opposition to the middle finger (after pollicization), otherwise thumb cutout.
- **Pressure points:**
  Palmar side: forearm to palm.
  Dorsal side: firm pad at distal forearm and at finger base joints (except thumb)
  Radial side: at the level of the 2nd metacarpal (plus 3rd metacarpal after pollicization) up to proximal forearm
  Ulnar side: distal forearm
- **Recommended materials** (Chap. 8):
  - Streif-Flex
  - Carbon brace
  - Deflector
  - Strap with Velcro fastener
  - Finger pad

2.2.6.3 Recurrence Treatment: Static-Progressive Wrist Extension Orthosis

If a recurrence develops despite orthotic treatment, or if the rigid orthosis cannot prevent a radial and/or palmar angulation in the wrist, a static-progressive orthotic treatment may be useful. Especially in children with TAR syndrome, a strong tendon-muscle pull can be observed, which pulls the wrist to the palmar and radial side (Fig. 2.33). Here, static-progressive orthoses with or without individual finger encasement can help (Fig. 2.34a, b). They are used both at night and as exercise orthoses for short intervals during the day. At night, the

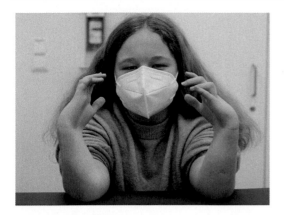

Fig. 2.33 13-year-old adolescent with TAR syndrome, after wrist erection. Recurrence tendency of the wrist to the palmar side with pronounced flexion contractures of the middle and ring fingers. (© Children's Hospital Wilhelmstift, with kind permission)

a strong extension of the fingers automatically occurs when the wrist is extended. Individual fingers with strong contractures can additionally be extended during the day using dynamic three-point finger extension orthoses (Fig. 2.34a, b) (Chap. 4).

▶ Whether this is feasible must be discussed with the patients and their parents in advance in order to determine both the time available and the motivation.

orthosis brings the wrist into a moderate, pain-free e xtension. At least 1–3 times a day, the orthosis is tightened to the pain threshold and worn for at least 10 to 30 minutes.

During the extension, the soft tissues on the dorsal side of the wrist are compressed. Therefore, the orthotic material must be "raised" there to guide the soft tissues (Chap. 8). A gencrous removal of the material is not advisable due to the changed soft tissue structure. If the fingers have flexion contractures, they are included in the orthosis. The fingers are placed into their guide without pressure and in wrist flexion, as

Static-Progressive Wrist Extension Orthosis
- **Hand position in the orthosis:**
  The hand and fingers rest in relaxed flexion in the orthosis, the wrist is extended as far as possible towards the ulnar side.
- **Orthosis coverage:**
  Free space circularly around the wrist
  The forearm is encased circularly or dorsally with wide straps to ensure stability during the extension in the orthosis.
  On the proximal forearm, the orthosis is as long as possible on the radial and ulnar sides without restricting movement, therefore usually a few

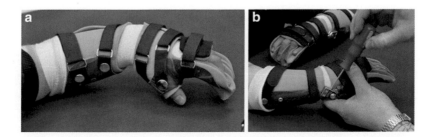

Fig. 2.34 a The same adolescent with static-progressive wrist extension orthosis for erecting the wrist dorsally and ulnarly. In addition, the middle finger joints are extended in the individual finger encasement—splint from the ulnar side. **b** Static-progressive wrist extension orthosis from the radial side, the extension is tightened to the pain threshold, the strong extension of the wrist intensifies the extension on the contracted fingers. (© Children's Hospital Wilhelmstift, with kind permission)

centimeters longer on the ulnar side to achieve maximum leverage.

The hand and thumb are encased circularly to prevent evasive movements during extension.

The fingers receive individual encasement from the palmar side, which also compensates for different contractures. A dorsal pressure pad on the finger base joints keeps the fingers in the orthosis.

- **Pressure points:**
  Palmar side: forearm and palm.
  Dorsal side: firm pad over the entire length from the distal to the proximal forearm and on the back of the hand, a pad over the finger base joints
  Radial side: the entire forearm, the hand at the 2nd metacarpal bone; the thumb guide expands the pressure point; with individual finger encasement the pressure point is extended distally to the tip of the index finger
  Ulnar side: distal forearm
- **Recommended materials** (Chap. 8):
  - Streif-Flex
  - Carbon brace
  - Deflector
  - Strap with Velcro fastener
  - Finger pad
  - Static dynamic joint

Caution:
If the wrist is extended in the orthosis, there is automatically a stronger extension of the fingers in the orthosis, therefore they must be encased in a relaxed position in wrist flexion. The edges at the level of the dorsal wrist must be generously "raised" due to the soft tissue displacement (Chap. 8)

2.2.6.4 Dynamic Finger Extension Orthoses

To specifically treat individual finger middle joints (Fig. 2.35a), the therapy can be intensified with dynamic finger extension orthoses (Fig. 2.35b). These splints are worn several times a day for 10–30 min. The pressure points are located on the palmar side at the base joint and at the finger middle phalanx. Dorsally, the counter pressure is at the level of the finger base phalanx. The spring system of the orthosis pushes the middle joint into extension (Chaps. 4 and 8).

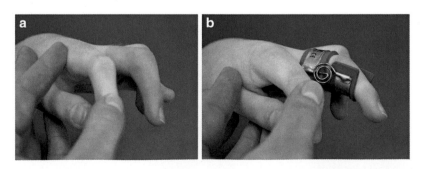

Fig. 2.35 **a** Pronounced flexion contractures of the finger middle joints 3 and 4. **b** Treatment with a dynamic finger extension orthosis from RUCK. (© Children's Hospital Wilhelmstift, with kind permission)

2.2.7 Treatment Examples Depending on Development and Therapy Status

2.2.7.1 Preoperative Situation

This little boy was presented to us at the age of 7 months (Fig. 2.36a–c). In addition to a bilateral radial longitudinal reduction defect type 4, he has right thumb aplasia and left thumb hypoplasia. Both forearms are shortened and the ulnas are curved. The fingers show extension on contractures in the base joints and severe flexion contractures in the middle joints. Intensive manual stretching of the hand and finger joints as well as splint treatment with thermoplastic splints to stretch the wrists began on this day. At the age of 12 months, the previous splints were replaced by forearm splints with finger encasement (Fig. 2.16a, b).

Through daily manual treatment by the mother and nightly splint or orthosis therapy, the wrists and fingers can be stretched and thus the active mobility is significantly improved (Fig. 2.37a, b), which promotes the child's development, independence, and dexterity.

2.2.7.2 Conservative treatment in severe forms of RLD

In this little girl conservative therapy has proven successful. Surgical measures are probably not possible, as they would deprive the girl of the ability to reach her mouth with her right hand (Figs. 2.17a, b and 2.38). Through growth and manual treatment of all fingers, the shoulders, and the right wrist, the girl can extend and flex

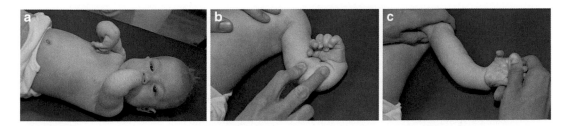

Fig. 2.36 **a** 8-month-old boy with RLD on both sides, right thumb aplasia, left thumb hypoplasia, and bilateral finger flexion contractures. **b** Active extension of the fingers is not possible, the hand lies on the forearm, active movements to the ulnar side are only possible to a minimal degree. **c** The hand can only be stretched passively with a lot of force. The strong flexor tendon and muscle pull can be seen in the palm. A lot of force is needed to stretch the wrist to the ulnar side. (© Children's Hospital Wilhelmstift, with kind permission)

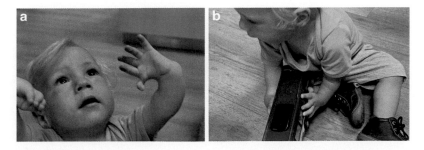

Fig. 2.37 **a** Same boy at the age of 18 months after 7 months of treatment with forearm orthoses with finger encasement and intensive manual treatment by the mother. The active mobility of the wrist to the ulnar and dorsal side as well as the finger mobility have significantly improved. **b** The flexor muscles and tendons have become more elastic through the treatment and allow an active opening of the hand. (© Children's Hospital Wilhelmstift, with kind permission)

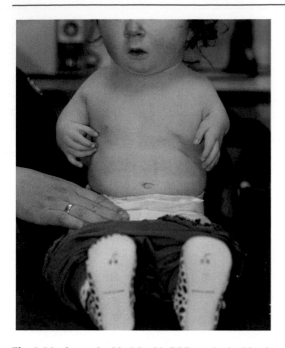

Fig. 2.38 9-month-old girl with RLD on both sides in TAR syndrome, missing right forearm, very short fused upper and lower arm on the left, hypoplastic thumbs and limited finger mobility on both sides. (© Children's Hospital Wilhelmstift, with kind permission)

her fingers more actively and bring her wrist into a significantly better ulnar deviation after 12 months of treatment (Fig. 2.39b). Bimanual activities have become possible (Fig. 2.39a), the gripping radius has improved mainly through the stretching of the radial soft tissues of the right wrist. Since the 9th month of life, in addition to manual treatment, therapy with night splints for stretching the right wrist to the ulnar and dorsal side has been carried out (Fig. 2.2).

For a child with this severe malformation, the enabling of bimanual activities and a slightly increased range of motion is a big step towards independence.

2.2.7.3 Pre- and postoperative situation

In this patient, we show the preoperative situation at the age of 9 months, the postoperative situation, and, after many years of recurrence treatment, the situation at the age of 13 years. Preoperatively, there is a bilateral radial longitudinal reduction defect with complete radius aplasia and thumb aplasia as well as finger flexion contractures. Surgical interventions:

- Straightening of the wrists using a half-ring fixator,
- Radialisation,
- Removal of K-wire and pollicization on the right and left hand.

In addition to many physical activities, the young man plays handball.

Preoperative situation at 9 months: radial longitudinal reduction defect type 4 with thumb aplasia and finger flexion contractures on both sides (Fig. 2.40a, b).

At the age of just under 3 years: after straightening of the wrist using a half-ring fixator, radialisation, removal of K-wire and pollicization at the right hand (Fig. 2.41a, b).

At the age of 5 years: after straightening of the wrists using a half-ring fixator, radialisation, removal of K-wire and pollicization at the right and left hand (Fig. 2.42a, b).

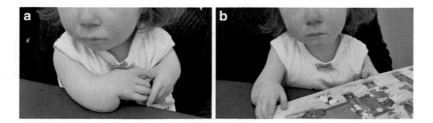

Fig. 2.39 **a** Same girl at the age of 21 months after 12 months of conservative treatment. Bimanual activities are possible. **b** The gripping radius has increased due to the stretched radial soft tissues of the right wrist. (© Children's Hospital Wilhelmstift, with kind permission)

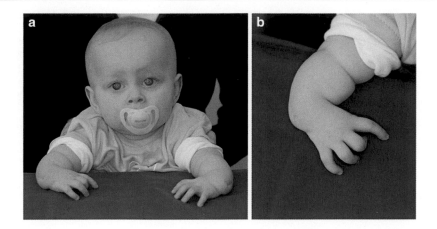

Fig. 2.40 a, b Patient at the age of 9 months, with RLD, thumb aplasia and finger flexion contractures on both sides. (© Children's Hospital Wilhelmstift, with kind permission)

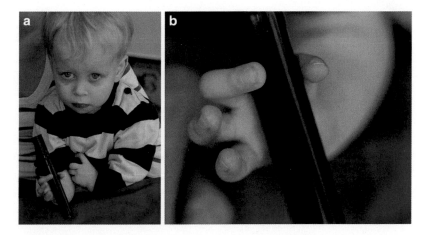

Fig. 2.41 a, b Patient at the age of just under 3 years, after wrist straightening and pollicization on the right. (© Children's Hospital Wilhelmstift, with kind permission)

At the age of 13 years: ongoing, consistent nightly splint therapy to prevent recurrences and to stretch the fingers with significant improvement of the finger flexion contractures (Fig. 2.43a, b).

It is important for the child's development to allow and promote all activities both pre- and postoperatively:

e.g. crawling, propping up (Fig. 2.44a, b), climbing (Fig. 2.44c), playing handball, learning a musical instrument. Many activities are also possible using aids, or be come easier with aids (Chap. 7), such as playing a musical instrument, riding a balance bike or bicycle.

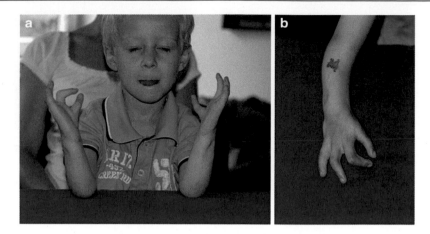

Fig. 2.42   a, b Patient at the age of 5 years, after wrist straightening and pollicization on both sides. (© Children's Hospital Wilhelmstift, with kind permission)

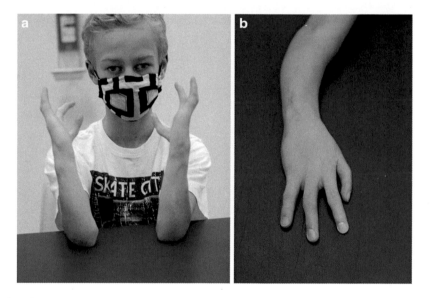

Fig. 2.43   a, b Patient at the age of 13 years, after wrist straightening and pollicization on both sides, as well as constant splint therapy to prevent recurrences and to stretch fingers 3–5. (© Children's Hospital Wilhelmstift, with kind permission)

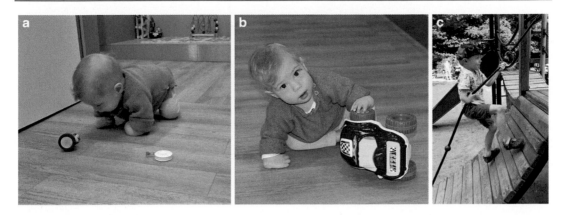

Fig. 2.44 **a** 14-month-old boy with RLD on both sides, thumb aplasia on the right, thumb hypoplasia on the left and finger flexion contractures on both sides (preoperative situation). The hands are angled 90° to the radial side next to the ulna, crawling is mainly done on the forearms over the ulnar sides. **b** The child often supports itself by the edge of the hand. **c** 5-year-old boy with RLD and thumb aplasia on the right, manual stretching of the wrist from the 8th month of life without surgical care. He pulls himself up with the healthy arm, the right arm stabilizes the climbing action, the rope is held in the interdigital grip. (© Children's Hospital Wilhelmstift, with kind permission)

References

Bayne LG, Kluge MS (1987) Long-term review of surgicaltreatment of radial deficiencies. J Hand Surg Am 12(2):169–79. https://doi.org/10.1016/s0363-5023(87)80267-8

Hülsemann W (voraussichtl. 2023) Handfehlbildungen im Kindes- und Jugendalter. In: Spies et al (Hrsg) Unterarm und Hand. Springer, Berlin

Thumb Hypoplasia and Thumb Aplasia

3

Contents

3.1 Clinical Picture

The **thumb hypoplasia** is a congenital under-development of the thumb ray, affecting all structures such as bones, muscles, and tendons. The extent of underdevelopment ranges from a reduction of the thumb to the absence of essential parts to the complete absence of the entire ray, the **thumb aplasia.**

The degrees of hypoplasia are classified according to Blauth (Fig. 3.1), in the modification by Manske.

- Grade I:
  Slimness of the thumb without clinical relevance. The intrinsic thenar musculature is slightly hypoplastic.
  Consequence: minor, possibly faster fatigue when painting or writing.
- Grade II:
  The thenar musculature is not regularly formed, the collateral ligaments of the metacarpophalangeal joint are unstable, the first interdigital fold and the hand skeleton are narrowed.

Consequences: the unstable collateral ligaments significantly reduce strength.
- Grade IIIA:
  In addition to the deficits of grade II, there are anomalies of the extrinsic musculature, an unstable saddle joint due to hypoplasia of the proximal first metacarpal, and a lack of intrinsic musculature (Chap. 1). The instability of the thumb significantly limits strength.
  Consequences: Overuse pain with adduction contracture.
- Grade IIIB:
  The proximal portion and thus the base of the first metacarpal is not formed and the functionally important saddle joint is missing (Fig. 3.1).
  Consequences: The thumb is largely non-functional. It cannot be used for gripping due to lack of stability. The interdigital grip is used as a substitute.
- Grade IV:
  The rudimentary thumb is only connected to the hand by skin, it floats (=floating thumb).
  Consequence: the thumb is completely non-functional.

M. Schelly and A.-L. Dunse, *Pediatric Hand Deformities in Occupational Therapy and Physical Therapy*,
https://doi.org/10.1007/978-3-662-68715-4_3

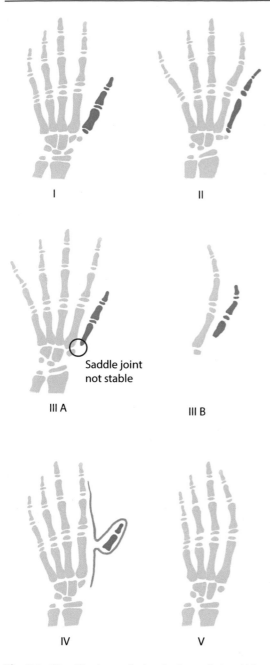

I   II

Saddle joint
not stable

III A   III B

IV   V

Fig. 3.1 Classification of thumb hypoplasia (After Blauth Blauth 1967, modified by Manske 1992. From Hülsemann presumably 2023)

- Grade V:
  Complete aplasia of the thumb ray, the scaphoid is reduced in size.

Thumb hypoplasia can occur in isolation or as part of a more complex malformation, for example, a radial longitudinal reduction defect (Chap. 2).

3.2   Treatment

After a clinical examination, depending on the severity of the thumb hypoplasia, an **operative therapy** is performed. From thumb hypoplasia grade IIIB onwards, pollicization of the index finger is considered the best method in Europe to construct a functioning thumb in one step. Often, it is difficult for parents to have the existing but non-functioning thumb removed and to decide on the index finger pollicization. Preoperatively, a functional analysis by occupational or physiotherapists can be useful for an externally existing but non-functioning thumb (Fig. 3.2a, b) to help parents in decision-making. If the thumb is completely omitted during gripping and only gripped in the side grip = interdigital grip, the finding corresponds to that of a non-existent thumb. In many cases, a rotation of the index finger develops into slight opposition and the second interdigital fold widens spontaneously (Fig. 3.2b). The index finger already starts to take over the function of the thumb. The hint at this adaptation can help parents in the decision to have the index finger surgically moved to the thumb position. Pollicization significantly expands the gripping possibilities. For example, precision and power grips only become possible after this procedure (Chap. 1).

3.2.1   Surgical Therapy

- Grade I:
  No surgical therapy necessary
- Grade II and IIIA:
  In cases of partially non-existent thenar muscles and instability of the thumb base joint due to collateral ligament insufficiency, both can be improved by **opponensplasty** by transposition of the flexor digitorum

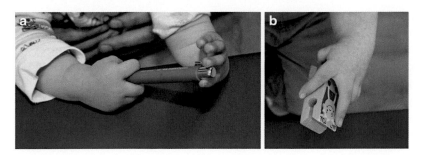

Fig. 3.2 **a** 16-month-old girl with thumb hypoplasia IIIB on the right and thumb aplasia due to radial longitudinal reduction defect on the left. Due to the severe thumb hypoplasia, the girl can only hold the pencil in the interdigital grip. The thumb of the right hand is completely omitted and has no function. **b** 2-year-old girl. Due to the non-functioning hypoplastic thumb, the interdigital grip has become the dominant gripping form. The index finger shows a slight opposition. (© Children's Hospital Wilhelmstift, with kind permission)

superficialis IV tendon. At the same time, the first interdigital fold is widened by a simple or double **Z-plasty** or a **rotation expansion flap** from the back of the hand.

- Grade IIIB, IV and V:

  In case of instability or non-existence of the thumb saddle joint, in most cases a **pollicization** is performed to achieve the best possible functional result. During pollicization, the hypoplastic thumb is resected. The index finger ray is shortened and placed in pronation and palmar abduction in the thumb position.

3.2.2 Surgical Techniques

3.2.2.1 Opponensplasty

The superficial flexor tendon of the ring finger (Flexor-digitorum-superficialis-IV-tendon = FDS 4) is detached at the ring finger, retracted proximally to the wrist, led around the FCR tendon, and transposed to the 1st metacarpal. One leg of the FDS tendon is pulled through a bone canal to the ulnar side and fixed with defined tension on the 1st metacarpal. Then both legs are inserted at the base of the proximal phalanx for stabilization of the collateral ligaments (Fig. 3.3). This allows circumduction, improves abduction and opposition, and stabilizes the thumb metacarpophalangeal joint.

3.2.2.2 Z-Plasty

A **Z-plasty** is a Z-shaped skin incision, where the skin flap with the subcutis is transposed to the opposite side and sutured. This extends the skin.

3.2.2.3 Rotational Flap Expansion

By mobilizing a dorsal skin flap from the back of the hand, skin is pulled into the interdigital fold, which is thus effectively expanded.

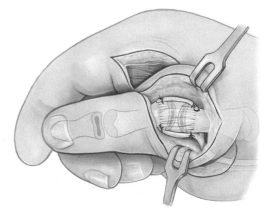

Fig. 3.3 The superficial flexor tendon of the ring finger was transposed to the 1st metacarpal. For stabilization of the metacarpophalangeal joint, one leg is augmented on the radial side and another, after being pulled through a bone canal, on the ulnar side to the collateral ligaments. (From Hülsemann expected 2023)

3.2.2.4 Pollicization

From a thumb hypoplasia grade IIIB onwards, the instability of the saddle joint and the expected shortness of the thumb at the end of growth are an indication for a **pollicization.** In the case of hypoplasia grade IV and V, it is the *only* option to improve the gripping function.

In pollicization, the following is done:

- the index finger is shortened by resecting the middle portion of its metacarpal,
- the index finger base joint becomes the new pseudo saddle joint, the former index finger proximal interphalangeal joint becomes the new thumb base joint (Fig. 3.4a, b),
- the metacarpal head is sutured in hyperextension with the joint capsule to avoid hyperextension at the level of the new saddle joint.
- the index finger is fixed in a 90 to 110° rotation on the base of the second metacarpal. Thus, no saddle joint with two degrees of freedom is formed as would be the case in a normal hand.

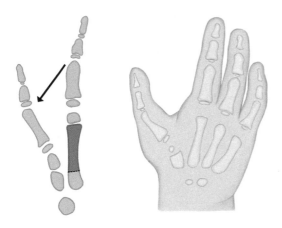

Fig. 3.4 a Illustration of pollicization = the transposition of the index finger to the thumb position. The index finger proximal interphalangeal joint becomes the new thumb metacarpophalangeal joint (red arrow), the metacarpophalangeal joint becomes the new pseudo saddle joint. The metacarpal of the index finger is significantly shortened by resecting the middle portion (red portion). **b** The index finger is fixed in a 90 to 110° rotation on the base of the second metacarpal. The new thumb is in 20 to 30° radial abduction and 40° palmar abduction and thus in opposition to the ring finger. (From Hülsemann expected 2023)

- the new thumb is positioned in 20 to 30° radial abduction and 40° palmar abduction and thus in opposition to the ring finger. The extensor tendon is shortened and the flexor tendons (M. flexor digitorum profundus/M flexor digitorum superficialis) are left to spontaneous shrinkage.

For the interossei, there are the following surgical options:

According to Buck-Gramcko:

- Both interosseous muscles are detached from their lateral slips and after the bony adjustment, they are sutured together again in their new shorter length. They are supposed to replace the non-existent M. abductor and M. adductor.

Due to the pronounced scar formation, this surgical technique was changed in some centers following the recommendation of Mennen:

- The interosseous muscles are not detached from their attachment, but are left to spontaneous shortening.

Extensors and flexors are not balanced due to spontaneous shrinkage after the operation, this is only completed after about 3–6 months. Knowing the surgical technique is important for the correct and effective postoperative treatment.

3.2.3   Postoperative Treatment

3.2.3.1 Postoperative Care for Opponensplasty

Immobilization in a forearm-palm-thumb cast for 4 weeks with wide wrapping of the 1st interdigital fold, followed by further immobilization in a thumb cast for 2 weeks. Subsequently, we recommend **manual therapy** two to three times per week to train the new gripping pattern: all opposition exercises, the thumb tip should reach all fingertips and then the base of the little finger (Chap. 1 /Kapandji-Index).

Intensive **scar treatment** begins in the sixth postoperative week (Chap. 7).

Manual Therapy

In the first four weeks, the thumb is continuously immobilized in a cast. During this time, the patient should be guided to the following exercises:

- active movement of fingers 2–5 into the small and large fist as well as the lumbrical grip, the focus should be on the ring finger,
- to prevent a flexion contracture due to scar traction: active and passive stretching of the ring finger into extension several times a day,
- with the unaffected hand, active flexion in the ring finger middle joint with simultaneous opposition of the thumb. This leads to a stimulation of the cognitive motor to better initiate the movement on the affected side.

After the end of the third week, occupational can begin. This should initially take place without load. The splint may only be removed during the exercise phases.

The focus is on:

- Initiation of active opposition: the patient performs a flexion with the ring finger and imagines the opposition of the thumb. Gradually, the imagination becomes an assistive and then an active movement.
- Active flexion in both ring finger middle joints and simultaneous opposition of the thumb on both sides,
- active mobilization of the wrist,
- scar treatment to counteract adhesions,
- active initiation of radialduction and palmarduction,
- exercise of the physiological use of the thumb, opposition to the fingertips of fingers 2–5 and eventually to the base of the little finger.

From the 7th postoperative week, the splint only needs to be worn in situations of stress or danger. The following exercises can now be included in the treatment:

- load-free active and passive opposition exercises,
- holding and gripping exercises with light objects,
- active exercise of fine coordination,
- to support the opposition, an opponens loop can be used, for example with an NRX tape (Chap. 8) (Fig. 3.5a, b).

From the 10th postoperative week, full mobilization without restrictions is possible:

- isometric strengthening exercises in abduction and opposition,
- dynamic strengthening exercises in abduction and opposition,
- continued exercise of fine motor skills and fine coordination.

▶ In addition, the handedness of the child should taken into account during postoperative care. If the operated hand is the dominant hand, exercises for graphomotor skills should be started early.

3.2.3.2 Postoperative Care for Pollicization

Immobilization of the thumb in abduction and opposition to the ring and middle finger for 10 days in a bandage. From about the 7th to 10th postoperative day, a thumb cast provides additional immobilization for another four weeks.

From the fifth postoperative week, intensive **scar treatment** is carried out several times a day.

Manual therapy begins immediately after the surgical control five weeks postoperatively and takes place two to three times a week, to train the new gripping pattern.

Depending on the findings, a **splint treatment** with a thermoplastic splint is necessary. This treatment counteracts scar shrinkage and thus the narrowing of the 1st interdigital fold and stabilizes the desired opposition position.

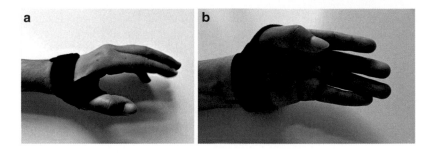

Fig. 3.5 a Application of an opponens loop 7 weeks after opponensplasty for assistive exercise of opposition. This loop (NRX tape) supports the patient by keeping the thumb in palmarduction. **b** View from the palmar side, the thumb is in palmarduction in front of the index finger, so that fine motor exercises can be performed with the patient. © Children's Hospital Wilhelmstift, with kind permission

Immobilization

The new thumb must be wrapped in abduction and opposition to the middle and ring finger for five weeks. (Fig. 3.6a–d). From about the 10th postoperative day, after a significant reduction in swelling, a small cast splint on the dorsal side of the entire thumb ray supports the immobilization. The bandage is left in place for another 3–4 weeks after the cast splint is applied and only then removed.

▶ Tip The soft tissues of the first interdigital fold swell postoperatively. The strongest tendency to swell is observed in the first four to six days. Due to the extent of the surgical procedure, tension blisters (Fig. 3.7) can occur due to superficial circulatory disorders on the mobilized skin flap. The hand must be kept still, especially in the first 10 days after the operation, and during the day it must be tied up at heart level, e.g. by a loop. This allows the child to move and play with the

non-operated hand. It is minimally restricted and the operated hand is protected and elevated.

After the fifth postoperative week and removal of the bandage, a control examination must be carried out before the first treatment:

- Trophicity of the scar,
- Soft tissue swelling,
- Position of the thumb,
- Passive and active range of motion of the thumb base and end joint,
- Status quo of the gripping forms used by the child.

The manual therapy and a possible splint treatment are based on the surgical therapy and the postoperative findings.

The **scar treatment** after pollicization poses a challenge. Scars after pollicization tend to be extremely firm and to show contractures.

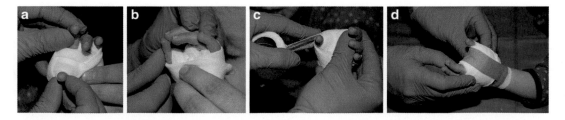

Fig. 3.6 a–d The new thumb is wrapped in the best possible opposition and abduction after the operation. The base and end joint must not be overstretched. (© Children's Hospital Wilhelmstift, with kind permission)

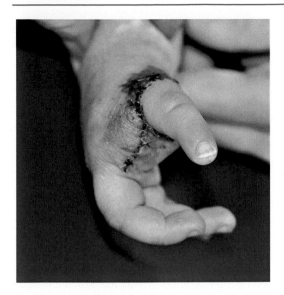

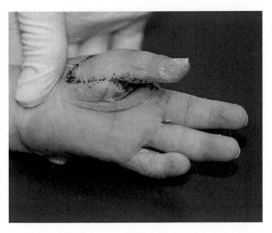

Fig. 3.8 The thumb is in adduction five weeks postoperatively due to insufficiently wide wrapping. (© Children's Hospital Wilhelmstift, with kind permission)

Fig. 3.7 12th day postoperatively. The hand is swollen, small tension blisters have formed. (© Children's Hospital Wilhelmstift, with kind permission)

Scar treatment starts from the fifth postoperative week after removal of the plaster bandage. The skin is very dry and crusted at this time (Fig. 3.8). Applying a fat cream several times a day supports the regeneration of the skin and facilitates the removal of the crusts.

The scar mobilization is carried out several times a day (e.g. after each diaper change) on and next to the scar with circular movements. The new thumb is held in the best possible opposition and abduction with the holding hand. Overextension of the thumb base joint must be absolutely prevented.

▶ The strong scar pull after pollicization is a result of the extensive operation and the large-scale preparation of the skin soft tissues.

In addition to scar massage, manual stretching to widen the first interdigital fold is essential to counteract adduction contractures (Figs. 3.8, 3.9 and 3.10).

To stretch the first interdigital fold:

● the therapist grasps the child's hand from the ulnar edge of the hand, so that he can fix the wrist and 3rd metacarpal well,
● with the other hand, the 2nd metacarpal is grasped and stretched towards palmar flexion (Fig. 3.9).
● The therapist's thumb is on the palmar side at the level of the new MP joint, the index finger is on the dorsal side distal to the MP joint, and the middle finger is on the dorsal side proximal to the MP joint.

▶ Warning The therapist must hold the thumb in opposition during manipulation and fix both the neo-saddle joint and the thumb base joint to prevent pushing the thumb into radialduction or overextending the base joint, as this would cause the thumb to lose much of its opposition.
The child is allowed to support itself, crawl, etc. and this should not be prevented.

The **Manual Therapy** starts parallel to scar treatment.

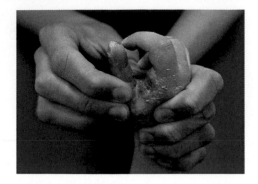

Fig. 3.9 3-year-old boy after pollicization. The thumb is in insufficient abduction 5 weeks after the operation. Scar massage and stretching of the first interdigital fold are performed by strong traction and manipulation. A hyperextension in the base joints must be prevented by the therapist's fixation. (© Kinderkrankenhaus Wilhelmstift, with kind permission)

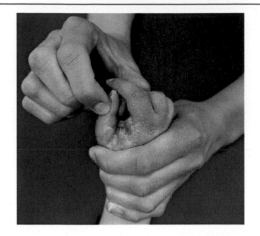

Fig. 3.11 5 weeks postoperatively after removal of the bandage. The skin is dry, the scars are red, and the passive mobility of the base joint is limited. The thumb base joint is stretched into flexion. (© Kinderkrankenhaus Wilhelmstift, with kind permission)

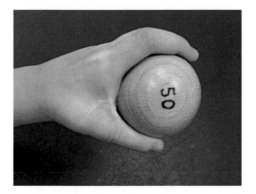

Fig. 3.10 Result 2 years postoperatively. The stretching and splint treatment were successful. The child can also grasp very large objects. (© Kinderkrankenhaus Wilhelmstift, with kind permission)

and thus presses the thumb base joint into flexion.

Actively (Figs. 3.12 and 3.13):

- the new thumb is held by the therapist's holding hand from the radial side in a good opposition, with the therapist's thumb lying palmar proximal to the thumb base joint,
- the child performs an active flexion in the thumb base joint. For this, it may need a small incentive, such as tickling a stuffed animal.

To improve flexion in the **thumb base joint** (Fig. 3.11), the following passive and active movements are performed.

Passively:

- the thumb is fixed by the therapist's holding hand from the ulnar side in a good opposition position, with the therapist's thumb lying palmar proximal to the thumb base joint. The remaining fingers encircle the thumb dorsally in a good palmar flexion.
- The index finger of the other hand is placed dorsal proximal to the child's thumb end joint

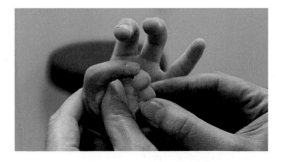

Fig. 3.12 After the passive stretch, the child is guided to actively practice the newly gained range of motion. To initially achieve targeted control of the base joint, the hand must be held. (© Kinderkrankenhaus Wilhelmstift, with kind permission)

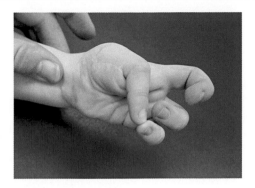

Fig. 3.13 2 years after pollicization. The child can optimally flex the thumb base joint. Opposition to the little finger pad is possible. This corresponds to a Kapandji score of 6. (© Kinderkrankenhaus Wilhelmstift, with kind permission)

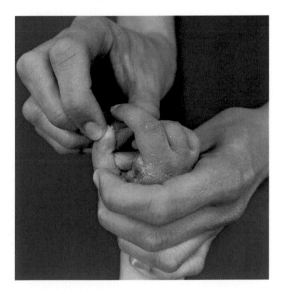

Fig. 3.14 Passive stretching of the thumb distal joint into flexion. (© Kinderkrankenhaus Wilhelmstift, with kind permission)

To improve the flexion in the **thumb distal joint** (Fig. 3.14), the following passive and active movements are performed.

Passively:

- the thumb is fixed in good opposition by the therapist as described above,
- the holding hand slides a little further distally, so that the therapist's thumb lies palmar proximal to the thumb distal joint,

- in this position, the thumb distal joint is stretched into flexion over the holding thumb of the therapist (Fig. 3.14).

Actively:

- the child's neo-thumb is fixed radially by the therapist in good opposition at the level of the first phalanx,
- the therapist's thumb is palmar, proximal to the thumb distal joint (Fig. 3.15),
- the child is now asked to flex the thumb distal joint (Fig. 3.15). The therapist fixes the base joint to initiate selective flexion in the thumb distal joint. This can also be done by tickling a stuffed animal.

All these exercises should be performed several times a day to train the mobility and strength of the new thumb and to form the neo-thumb in the motor cortex of the brain (Fig. 3.16).

The opposition position is important for the best possible functional use of the new thumb. Children must be motivated through various materials to exercise diverse gripping forms with the thumb, e.g., precision grip, penny grip, key grip, three-point grip, and bilateral activities (Fig. 3.17a–c). The lateral grip/interdigital grip, which the children have internalized before the

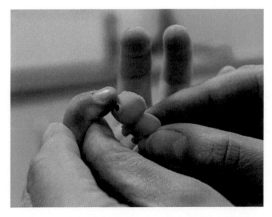

Fig. 3.15 After the passive stretch has taken place, the child is motivated to practice active control. To initially achieve targeted control of the distal joint, the hand must be held. (© Kinderkrankenhaus Wilhelmstift, with kind permission)

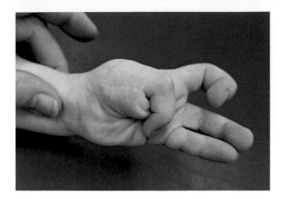

Fig. 3.16 2 years postoperatively. The flexion in the base and distal joint is end-range, opposition to the little finger base joint is possible. This corresponds to a Kapandji score of 10. (© Kinderkrankenhaus Wilhelmstift, with kind permission)

operation, must be retrained. If the child does not use the thumb during the course of treatment, the middle and ring fingers (possibly also the little finger) can be wrapped together using tape (Fig. 3.18a, b). Using the new thumb stimulates the sensorimotor cortex and thus promotes the conscious execution of thumb opposition. In addition, wrist extension should be practiced with the child.

▶ In addition, the handedness of the child should be taken into account during the follow-up treatment. This may have been influenced by the long period of immobilization. Often it takes a few days until the children

use the affected hand again in everyday life. If the operated hand is the dominant hand, exercises for graphomotor skills should be started early.

Sensory stimulations to improve the perception of the new thumb and the sense of touch can be done, for example, with a brush, paintbrush, vibration, sponge, or by treasure hunting in warm or cold rapeseed, cherry pits, pebble baths, and playing in the sand.

Various age-appropriate gripping exercises and bimanual activities to improve the physiological use and abduction can be carried out with toy blocks, pegboards, card games, board games, clay, beads, play dough, craftwork, large balls, stacking cups, large marbles for the marble run, and pouring games with various sized containers.

If the child continues to use the interdigital grip, the fingers should be solidarized. This takes away the child's ability to fall back into old gripping patterns. If the fixation of the base phalanges is not sufficient, the fingers can also be solidarized at the level of the middle phalanges. The solidarization can be maintained for several hours or even the whole day. The fixation can be done, for example, with a Buddy Loop® (Fig. 3.18a, b), NRX®-Tape or Peha-Haft® (Chap. 8). Over time, the precision grip becomes automatic and the child gives up the interdigital grip, the precision grip is used securely.

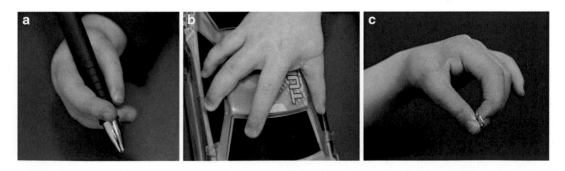

Fig. 3.17 a, b Neo-thumb 7 months post-op. The fine grip for holding a pen is possible, but still clumsy. Even large objects can be grasped. The gripping strength is further strengthened. **c** The finest grips can be executed purposefully with the thumb. (© Children's Hospital Wilhelmstift, with kind permission)

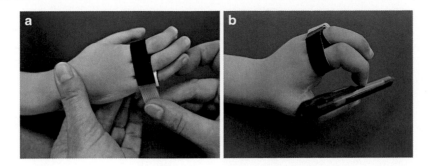

Fig. 3.18 a, b Fingers 3–5 are fixed with a Buddy Loop® to prevent the interdigital grip. The child should constantly practice the use of the precision grip in everyday life. (© Children's Hospital Wilhelmstift, with kind permission)

Splint Treatment

If the first interdigital fold is scarred and narrowed and/or the thumb is in insufficient opposition (Fig. 3.19), the condition can be significantly improved by a splint.

Before the construction of the thermoplastic splint, the scars are loosened as much as possible by shifting the skin layers and the thumb is massaged into the desired position (20 to 30° radial abduction/40° palmar abduction). The stretching takes time to significantly improve the position and create a good starting position for an optimal splint fit.

- The holder fixes fingers 3–5 and the proximal forearm.

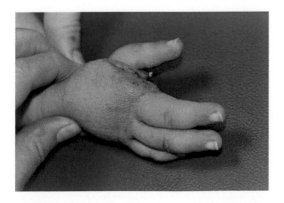

Fig. 3.19 5 weeks after pollicization. The neo-thumb is located too much in the plane of the hand with too little opposition to the middle and ring finger. The scar pull is pronounced and pulls the thumb into adduction. (© Children's Hospital Wilhelmstift, with kind permission)

- The child's elbow is placed on a support for better stabilization, fingers 3–5 are slightly pulled distally and dorsally to prevent the wrist from twisting and to position the wrist in 20–30° extension.
- To ensure the splint fits well and does not slip, it covers the entire back of the hand up to the distal forearm, the wrist, the edge of the hand, and the thumb.
- It is modeled from the dorsal side deep into the first interdigital fold and to the palmar side of the first metacarpal bone and additionally from the dorsal side around the first metacarpal bone to the thumb base (Fig. 3.21a, b).

Pressure is applied during the modeling process:

- on the palmar proximal side of the thumb base joint (green arrow),
- on the palmar proximal side of the middle finger base joint (yellow arrow),
- on the dorsal thumb base (blue arrow).

Simultaneously
- the entire thumb ray is led into opposition to the middle and ring fingers (Fig. 3.20) (black arrow).

This positions the thumb in the best possible abduction and opposition to the middle and ring fingers and prevents hyperextension in the thumb base joint.

The edge of the hand is enclosed by the splint to prevent the hand from deviating to the

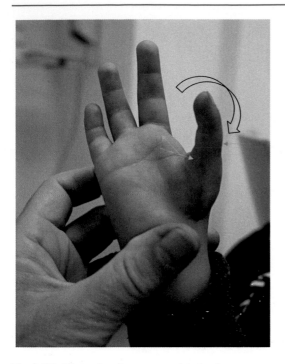

Fig. 3.20 The colored arrows point to the pressure points that need to be considered in the splint. The black arrow shows the movement of the thumb into opposition during the making of the splint. (© Children's Hospital Wilhelmstift, with kind permission)

ulnar side. Padding the splint on the palmar side around the thumb and the base joints of fingers 3–5 is useful to counteract pressure points caused by the retraction tendency due to scar tension (Fig. 3.21a, b).

The splint must be able to be opened at the level of the first metacarpal bone on the palmar side to facilitate putting it on, to not compress the blood vessels, and to leave additional room in case of swelling after hand therapeutic measures. Depending on the scar tension, the splint is worn for the first weeks over 12 to 20 hours, then for at least 3 more months at night. If scar treatment with silicone is necessary, this is done through a thin, elastic silicone film that optimally adapts to the small hand or through a silicone gel (Chap. 6). In some cases, a silicone pad

made of HTV silicone is advisable (Chap. 6). A tubular bandage under the splint protects the delicate skin of the children (Chap. 8). When treating with silicone gel, it should be frequently replaced to prevent skin irritation.

Forearm Splint after Pollicization
- **Hand and finger position in the splint:**
  Hand 1: Fingers 3–5 are pulled distally and dorsally.
  Hand 2: fixes the forearm and the elbow.
- **Splint coverage:**
  Approximately 2/3 of the circumference of the forearm and hand are enclosed. Complete enclosure on the dorsal side.
  The palm is modeled, the "new" thumb ray is encased up to the end joint, the edge of the hand is enclosed.
- **Pressure points:**
  Palmar side: palm, base joints of the middle finger and the neo-thumb, distal forearm
  Dorsal side: back of the hand and distal forearm, "new" first metacarpal and "new" thumb base phalanx Radially: "new" thumb pad
  Ulnarly: edge of the hand
  Caution: Prevent hyperextension in the base joints of the middle finger and the neo-thumb
- **Recommended materials:**
  – Thermoplastic material 2.0 mm
  – Tubular bandage 2.5 or 5 cm wide (Chap. 8)
  – Velcro strap
  – Fleece strap
  – Edge padding (Chap. 8)
  – Possibly padding between the splint edges (Chap. 8)

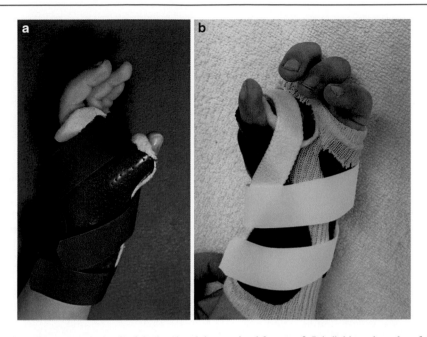

Fig. 3.21 a The splint covers the back of the hand and the proximal forearm. **b** It is led into the palm of the hand and around the neo-tumb from the dorsal side to the palmar side to splint it in the best possible abduction and opposition. The edge of the hand is enclosed to prevent it from deviating to the ulnar side. The splint is open on the palmar side at the first metacarpal bone to allow for swelling. (© Children's Hospital Wilhelmstift, with kind permission)

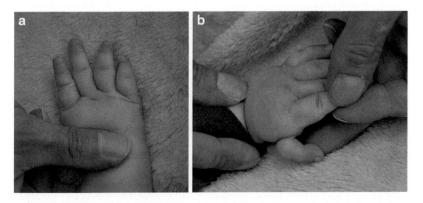

Fig. 3.22 a, b 9-month-old boy with right thumb aplasia and left Blauth IV thumb hypoplasia. (© Children's Hospital Wilhelmstift, with kind permission)

Caution:
When modeling the splint into opposition, the new thumb easily falls into adduction if the first interdigital fold is not simultaneously stretched. During the stretching of the first interdigital fold, the thumb must be pressed to the dorsal side proximal to the thumb base joint and the thumb base phalanx must be stretched palmarly to prevent hyperextension in the thumb base joint.

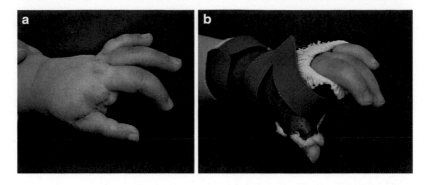

Fig. 3.23 **a** 2-year-old boy. 5 weeks after removal of the hypoplastic thumb and pollicization of the left index finger. **b** Due to scar traction and to optimize the position of the neo-thumb, a splint was fitted. The thumb is in the best possible abduction and opposition in the splint. (© Children's Hospital Wilhelmstift, with kind permission)

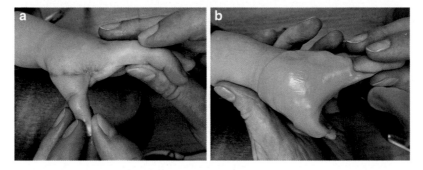

Fig. 3.24 **a** The scar is somewhat sunken, hardened, and barely movable. **b** An impression is taken with two-phase silicone to make an HTV silicone pad. In doing so, the neo-thumb is placed in the best possible abduction and opposition to the middle finger. (© Kinderkrankenhaus Wilhelmstift, with kind permission)

3.2.4   Treatment Example

9-month-old boy with right thumb aplasia and a left Blauth IV thumb hypoplasia (Fig. 3.22a, b).

The index finger was pollicized on both sides: at almost two years of age on the left side (Fig. 3.23a) and at two and a half years of age on the right side.

Five weeks after the pollicization on the left, a wound and position control was carried out. The parents were instructed in scar treatment, the occupational therapy took place intensively 2 to 3 times a week for several weeks. The boy received a thermoplastic splint, which splints the thumb in an optimal opposition and abduction position overnight (Fig. 3.23b).

Five months postoperatively, the thumb is in the desired opposition and abduction position.

Since the surgical scar continued to pull strongly (Fig. 3.24a), an impression was taken with two-phase silicone and an HTV silicone pad was made (Fig. 3.24b). In addition, the dimensions of the hand were taken for the manufacture of a compression glove.

In order for the HTV silicone pad to have a maximum effect (Fig. 3.25a), a compression glove is also made, which presses the pad tightly against the scar. A sewn-in zipper makes it easier to pull the glove over the pad. (Fig. 3.25b). The combination of pad and glove is worn overnight.

After four months of silicone and compression treatment, the scar is soft, elastic, and faded (Fig. 3.26).

The same boy at the age of three years after bilateral pollicization. The scars on the right

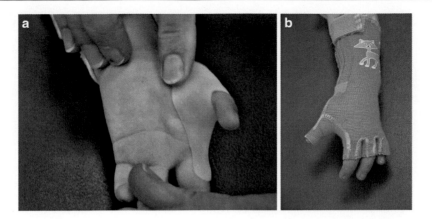

Fig. 3.25 **a** The HTV silicone pad is placed over the thumb into the first interdigital fold. All scars are covered by the pad. The pad guides the neo-thumb into the desired abduction and opposition. **b** A custom-made compression glove presses the pad tightly against the skin, allowing the pad to fully unfold its effect. (© Kinderkrankenhaus Wilhelmstift, with kind permission)

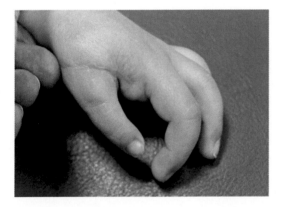

Fig. 3.26 2 ½-year-old boy. After four months of silicone and compression treatment, the scar is soft, elastic, and faded. (© Kinderkrankenhaus Wilhelmstift, with kind permission)

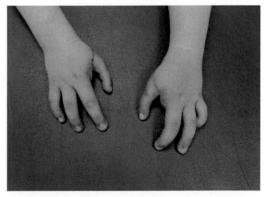

Fig. 3.27 Right hand 7 months and left hand 15 months postoperatively. The neo-thumbs are in a good abduction and opposition to the middle fingers. On the right hand, the scars are still in the remodeling phase. On the left, they are already soft and elastic. (© Kinderkrankenhaus Wilhelmstift, with kind permission)

hand are still remodeling 7 months postoperatively. The scars on the left hand are soft and elastic. The neo-thumbs are in a good abduction and opposition position (Fig. 3.27). The neo-saddle joints are stable.

Precision grips (Fig. 3.28a, b) as well as power grips (Chap. 1) are performed using the "new" thumbs. The handlebars of the balance bike are securely held with both hands and small cups are securely held in one hand with a power grip. The Kapandji index (Chap. 1) can be performed up to 6 on both sides. The hands can easily enclose a round object of 3 cm individually (Fig. 3.28c).

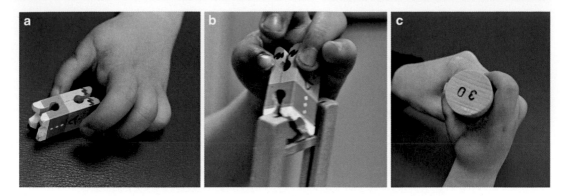

Fig. 3.28 a–c Precision and power grips can be performed using the "new" thumbs. (© Kinderkrankenhaus Wilhelmstift, with kind permission)

References

Blauth W (1967) The hypoplastic thumb. Arch Orthop Unfallchir 62:225–246

Hülsemann W (voraussichtl 2023) Handfehlbildungen im Kindes- und Jugendalter.In: Spies et al (Hrsg) Unterarm und Hand. Springer, Berlin

Manske PR, McCarroll HR (1992) Reconstruction of the congenitally deficient thumb. Hand Clin 8:177–196

Camptodactyly and Multiple Finger Flexion Contractures

4

Contents

Camptodactyly and multiple finger flexion contractures occur in various degrees and manifestations. They can affect one or more fingers on one or both hands.

They often occur in isolation, but can also be part of a complex malformation or a syndromal disease.

Camptodactyly and multiple flexion contractures, like the thumb-in-palm deformity, are classified as dysplasias. Dysfunctional cells lead to movement restrictions of the finger joints already during pregnancy and further growth.

4.1 Clinical Picture

The term camptodactyly comes from the Greek: kampto = I bend and daktylos = finger and refers to a flexion contracture of the middle joint of fingers 2 to 5. The little finger of one or both hands is most commonly affected, less often another finger (Fig. 4.1a, b). Camptodactyly most often appears in infancy as an early form = infantile form and less frequently, in less than 20%, as a late form = juvenile form in prepuberty.

Usually, the flexion malposition slowly increases during the child's growth, but can also deteriorate rapidly during a growth spurt. In rare cases, the flexion contracture remains stable.

The exact pathogenesis is unknown and appears to be multifactorial.

Possible causes include

- altered, shortened or incompletely developed superficial flexor tendons (FDS),
- lumbricals inserting in the wrong place (Chap. 1),
- thickened Cleland and Grayson ligaments.

As a result, it is likely that

- weakened extensor aponeuroses (Chap. 1),
- shortened palmar skin (Fig. 4.2a),
- shortened middle joint capsules occur.

The flexion contracture of the middle joint is often compensated by hyperextension in the base joint (Fig. 4.2a, c).

Radiologically, the following typical bone changes can be seen in severe forms:

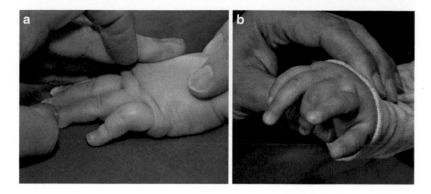

Fig. 4.1   **a** 10-month-old girl with camptodactyly of the little finger. **b** 11-month-old girl with camptodactyly of the middle finger. (© Children's Hospital Wilhelmstift, with kind permission)

- a narrowed and flattened base phalanx head,
- a palmar inclined base phalanx neck,
- a widening of the middle phalanx base (Fig. 4.2b).

The later the therapy begins, the more pronounced are both the bone changes and the shrinkage of the capsules. In some cases, a rotational malposition in the base joint develops as well (Fig. 4.2c). The compensatory hyperextension in the base joint intensifies, the palmar skin shortens further. During growth, intensive early therapy and stretchability of the fingers improve the bone structure (Netscher et al. 2015).

Even in infancy, a different resistance can be felt when passively extending the middle joint. If a hard stop is felt in the middle joint, this indicates more than just an imbalance between extensor and flexor tendons (Fig. 4.3a). On the other hand, an elastic joint and low resistance suggest an imbalance as the main cause (Fig. 4.3b). This can be checked with the tenodesis test (Fig. 4.3c, d).

▶ The **tenodesis test** is based on the anatomy of the flexors and extensors, whose tension is coordinated. When the wrist is flexed, the fingers passively extend. When the wrist is extended, the fingers passively flex.

This leads to the following in the examination for camptodactyly:

If the middle joint can be extended with a flexed wrist and/or base joint, this indicates a tendon shortening of the flexors.

This knowledge is important for manual therapy and splint treatment.

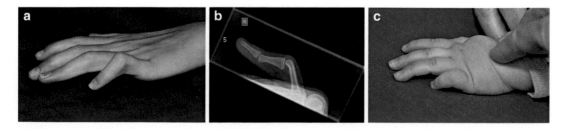

Fig. 4.2   **a** 11-year-old girl. Pronounced camptodactyly of the little finger with compensatory hyperextension in the base joint and wing-like shortening of the palmar skin. There is also a slight camptodactyly of the ring finger. **b** X-ray of a 13-year-old with subluxation position in the end joint and typical bone changes of the little finger middle joint: a narrowed and flattened base phalanx head, a palmar inclined neck and a widened middle phalanx base. **c** 10-month-old girl. Camptodactyly with rotational malposition of the little finger and hyperextension in the base joint. (© Children's Hospital Wilhelmstift, with kind permission)

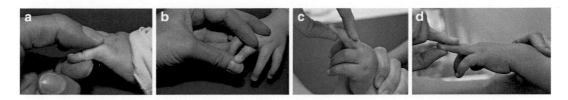

Fig. 4.3 **a** 10-month-old girl with camptodactyly of the little finger with a hard stop in the middle joint. **b** 14-month-old boy with camptodactyly of the middle finger. The middle joint can be fully extended passively. **c** 18-month-old boy with flexion contractures of fingers 2 to 5. The tenodesis test shows that there is a shortening of the flexors. When the wrist is overextended, full extension of the finger is not possible. **d** Full extensibility of the fingers with a flexed wrist. (© Children's Hospital Wilhelmstift, with kind permission)

4.2   Treatment

The treatment of infantile camptodactyly begins in infancy or early childhood, the treatment of the juvenile form immediately after diagnosis. In early childhood, the structures are still soft and elastic. This allows for much faster improvement and counteracts the shrinkage of the capsule-ligament apparatus.

Manual therapy and splint treatment are the first line of treatment. They should be carried out for at least one year. The compliance of parents and children is of great importance, especially when deciding on surgery, as the success of the operation strongly depends on the follow-up treatment (Foucher 2006). Surgery is only indicated after unsuccessful consistent conservative therapy and with a functionally limiting extension deficit of over 60°.

▶ The **earlier** and **more consistently** conservative treatment is carried out, the more promising the outcome!

4.2.1   Treatment Concept

Treatment proposal for children with infantile camptodactyly:

(The therapy for the juvenile form begins at point 4).

1. Manual therapy begins from the first days of life and is continuously carried on.

2. A static splint therapy with a thermoplastic splint or the so-called Glove-Splint is carried out from about the 8th month of life.
3. A dynamic finger splint can support the manual therapy during the day from about the second year of life.
4. An extended manual therapy by the parents and the child is carried out from about primary school age, supplemented by targeted active exercises to strengthen the muscles.
5. If, despite the treatment, surgery is necessary, the postoperative follow-up treatment must be intensive and take place after wound healing or after removal of the joint-fixing Kirschner wire.
6. In some cases, camptodactyly occurs on more than one finger of a hand or there are multiple flexion contractures on all three-jointed fingers of one or both hands. In these cases, intensive manual treatment and splint therapy are carried out. The splints must be made by orthopedic technicians due to the required individual finger enclosure.

▶ Treatment examples depending on the clinical picture and severity are presented at the end of the chapter.

In the initial phase, intensive therapy is required until there is a significant improvement in the extension deficit.

During growth spurts, it may be necessary to resume conservative treatment to prevent a recurrence. This information is given to patients and parents at the beginning of treatment. If the extension deficit worsens despite ongoing manual therapy, temporary re-splinting may be indicated.

▶ Therapeutic guidance begins in infancy and is reviewed and adjusted as necessary during growth.

4.2.2 Manual Therapy

Description using the example of a camptodactyly on the little finger.

4.2.2.1 Manual Stretching

In the **manual stretching** of the little finger, the wrist is first fixed with the holding hand in 20–30° extension to pre-stretch the flexor tendon (Fig. 4.4a). The therapist's holding hand fixes the wrist and the edge of the child's hand to prevent evasion. At the same time, the base joint of the finger to be treated is fixed to avoid hyperextension (Fig. 4.4b, c).

The index finger of the working hand is placed dorsally and proximally of the middle joint (Fig. 4.4b). It presses the affected finger towards the palmar side, so that the base joint is in flexion.

In this position, the middle joint automatically extends in a tendinogenic contracture as the flexor tendons relax. In the case of an arthrogenic cause, the joint remains firm (Fig. 4.4c).

In the next step, the thumb of the working hand supports the middle phalanx of the finger from the palmar side (Fig. 4.4c). The middle joint is stretched by the opposing pressure of the index finger and thumb (Fig. 4.4d). In this position, the affected finger is slowly extended in the base joint to the 0° position, which significantly increases the stretch on the middle joint (Fig. 4.4e). The finger is now held for a few seconds. This stretching is repeated.

▶ In the case of camptodactyly, manual stretching is important for therapeutic success and should be performed several times a day. It is useful to incorporate the stretching into everyday life and to perform it in infants and toddlers, after each diaper change, for example.

Caution:
During the entire stretching process, care must be taken not to put either the base or the end joint into hyperextension.

4.2.3 Glove-Splint, Splint and Orthosis Therapy

4.2.3.1 Glove-Splint

To support the manual stretching, splint therapy is started at about the 8th month of life. Splints

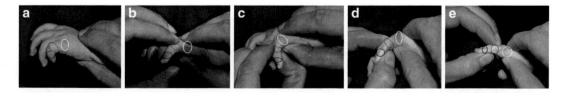

Fig. 4.4 a 7-month-old girl with camptodactyly of the little finger. The wrist is fixed in slight extension. **b** The holding hand also fixes the edge of the hand to prevent an evasive movement. **c** The index finger of the working hand presses the base joint into flexion from the dorsal side. The thumb supports the middle and end phalanx from the palmar side. The pressure point is focused on the palmar middle phalanx to avoid hyperextension in the end joint. **d** The middle joint is stretched by the opposing pressure of thumb and index finger. **e** The pressure on the middle joint is maintained and in this position the base joint is extended to the 0° position, thereby intensifying the stretching of the middle joint. Legend: Base joint—circled in white, middle joint—circled in blue, end joint—circled in red. (© Children's Hospital Wilhelmstift, with kind permission)

for infants and toddlers that are supposed to "only" encase one finger pose a great challenge to us as therapists:

- the splint should not slip,
- pressure points on the delicate, soft skin must be avoided
- and the removal of the splints by the child should be prevented.

To solve these problems, the **Glove-Splint** was developed for the treatment of camptodactylies and flexion contractures of individual fingers in infancy. It consists of a compression glove and a small thermoplastic splint (Fig. 4.5a–c). The compression glove holds the splint in the desired position with the sewn-on pocket and cushions the splint against the delicate skin. The splint only encases the joints of the finger to be treated, the other fingers remain free.

▶ The provision of a Glove-Splint is carried out in cooperation with a medical supply store— usually, orthopedic technicians take care of the production of the glove and the hand therapist adjusts the splint.

Manufacturing steps for the Glove-Splint
Description using the example of a supply for the little finger.
Several steps are needed to manufacture a Glove-Splint:

1. Measuring hand and forearm,
2. Drawing an outline,
3. Collecting additional information,
4. Manufacturing the small thermoplastic splint,
5. Photograph of the hand with and without splint,
6. Communication with the manufacturer.

▶ **Glove-Splint:** The glove is produced by companies that manufacture medical compression gloves. The cooperation takes place via a medial supply store (in Germany) (Chap. 8).

Making the Glove
For additional information, see measurement sheet (Table 4.1).

1. Taking measurements:

All measurements are taken loosely, without pulling on the skin (Fig. 4.6a, c). The only exception is the simultaneous treatment of scar tissue (Fig. 4.6b).

- Length measurements:
The cuff extends from the wrist to a maximum of half the forearm, in very small children up to the age of 18 months it is approx. 6 cm long. The intermediate measurement of the cuff is taken at about 3–4 cm from the distal end. The length of the palm is measured from the wrist to the interdigital fold/skin between the 3rd and 4th

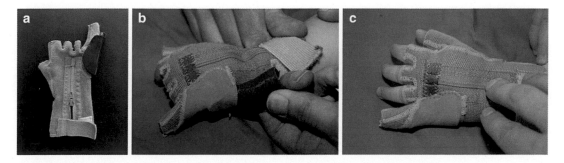

Fig. 4.5 **a** Compression stocking with sewn-on elastic pocket, next to it a small thermoplastic splint. **b** The small thermoplastic splint is inserted into the elastic pocket. **c** The splint fits snugly against the edge of the hand and the little finger. The glove can be put on more easily using the zipper. (© Children's Hospital Wilhelmstift, with kind permission)

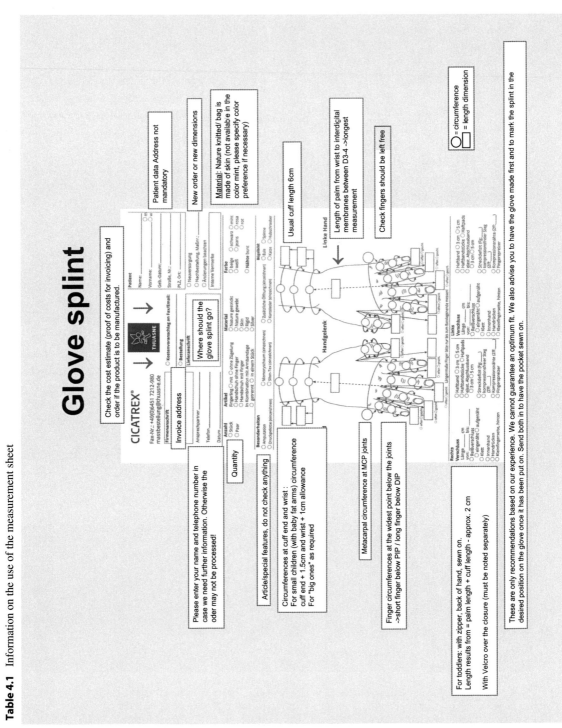

Table 4.1 Information on the use of the measurement sheet

Glove splint

Check the cost estimate (proof of costs for invoicing) and order if the product is to be manufactured.

Patient data Address not mandatory

New order or new dimensions

Material: Nature knitted/ bag is made of skin (not availabe in the color mint, please specify color preference if necessary)

Usual cuff length 6cm

Linke Hand

Length of palm from wrist to interdigital membranes between D3-4 ->longest measurement

Check fingers should be left free

Please enter your name and telephone number in case we need further information. Otherwise the oder may not be processed!

Article/special features, do not check anything

Circumferences at cuff end and wrist:
For small children (with baby fat arms) circumference
cuff end + 1.5cm and wrist + 1cm allowance
For "big ones" as required

Metacarpal circumference at MCP joints

Finger circumferences at the widest point below the joints
->short finger below PIP / long finger below DIP

For toddlers: with zipper, back of hand, sewn on.
Length results from = palm length + cuff length - approx. 2 cm

With Velcro over the closure (must be noted separately)

○ = circumference
▭ = length dimension

These are only recommendations based on our experience. We cannot guarantee an optimum fit. We also advise you to have the glove made first and to mark the splint in the desired position on the glove once it has been put on. Send both in to have the pocket sewn on.

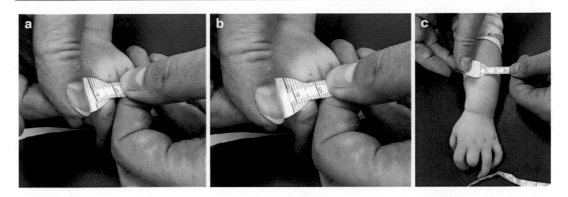

Fig. 4.6 a Measuring the index finger at skin level. **b** Measuring the index finger with tension. The difference in this child is 2mm. **c** Measuring the forearm at skin level at the desired end of the cuff. (© Children's Hospital Wilhelmstift, with kind permission)

finger (= longest measurement). The unaffected fingers are measured from the interdigital fold to the middle joints—not shorter, as the fabric pulls proximally. The thumb measurement extends from the depth of the irst interdigital fold to the thumb end joint, the measurement of the first interdigital fold from the depth of the first interdigital fold to the middle joint of the index finger. The little finger is measured in full extension to the fingertip. Depending on the flexion contracture of the little finger, it is additionally measured lengthwise from the dorsal and the palmar side. This is only necessary from a flexion contracture of 60°.

- Circumference measurements:

The circumferences of the forearm are measured at the wrist, the intermediate part and the end of the cuff (Fig. 4.6c). In very "chubby" children, the final measurement should be taken very loosely at skin level. The circumference of the middle hand is measured at the level of the base joints and the finger circumferences at their thickest point (usually slightly proximal to the middle joints) (Fig. 4.6a). The little finger requires an additional circumference measurement proximal to the end joint.

- Additional measurements:

To facilitate putting on the glove, a zipper sewn onto the back of the hand is recommended, which extends to the back of the hand (Fig. 4.5b, c). A Velcro fastener at the end of the

zipper cushions the slider and prevents scratching injuries (Fig. 4.5b). The zipper is sewn on, not sewn in. This protects the delicate skin from the pressure of the zipper.

Zipper length = palm length + cuff length − 2 cm

▶ All finger measurements are skin measurements. They are taken loosely, without tension. The only exception is simultaneous treatment of hypertrophic scars (Chap. 6).

Recommended materials:

- for the glove: Nature knitted
- for the pocket: Skin.
  This elastic and at the same time firm material allows the insertion of the splint and prevents it from slipping.

The production including the shipment takes about two weeks.

If the therapist is performing this type of care for the first few times, we recommend:

- First have the glove made.
- Mark the splint position on the worn glove.
- Send the marked glove and the splint back to the manufacturing company.

2. Making the outline drawing:

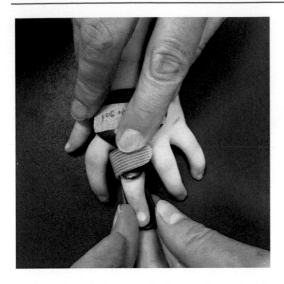

Fig. 4.7 The rein between the base and middle joint connects the dorsal splint with the palmar splint and is sewn in this position to the glove. This photo is important information for the splint manufacturer. (© Children's Hospital Wilhelmstift, with kind permission)

After taking measurements, an outline drawing of the hand is made. It serves:

- to control the dimensions,
- to transmit information to the manufacturer about the fit of the splint,
- to mark peculiarities or pathologies e.g. syndactylies, amputations,
- to mark the position of a rein (Fig. 4.7).

Additional information:

The manufacturer (Chap. 8) needs:

- Photos of the hand with (Fig. 4.7) and without a splint,
- Degree of flexion contracture of the finger to be treated,
- Desired position of a rein with photo (Fig. 4.7),
- Peculiarities or pathologies of the hand,
- Delivery address, delivery date, contact information for inquiries,
- Name of the patient,
- Material and color of the glove and the bag,
- Position of the zipper and the Velcro,
- Location of the bag opening (usually at the edge of the hand) (Fig. 4.5b),

- Photos are sent by email to the manufacturer in compliance with data protection regulations.

> **Caution:**
> Data protection: The parents must sign a consent form so that the child's data and photos can be sent to the glove manufacturer

Making the Thermoplastic Splint

For the small splint, which only splints the finger to be treated, thermoplastic material of 2.0 mm thickness is used for toddlers and infants. Unperforated material is recommended for better edge processing.

The splint encompasses:

- the entire little finger to the end of the metacarpal bone from the dorsal side (Fig. 4.8b),
- the little finger completely around the proximal phalanx (Fig. 4.8b),
- the palm up to the metacarpal bone of the ring finger, without obstructing the thenar muscles or the wrist (Fig. 4.8a).

It is important to ensure that all other joints apart from the little finger have free mobility. The wrist is given complete freedom of movement.

Important for the optimal production of the splint is quick work and a consistent holding of the hand to be treated. By holding the wrist in extension and fingers 2 to 4 under tension, the hand is in the optimal position for the splint maker (Fig. 4.9a).

The splint is gently formed around the finger and the edge of the hand, but not molded in. The delicate tissue is soft and would otherwise be exposed to too much pressure (Fig. 4.9b). During the modeling, the little finger is splinted by the splint maker from the palmar side and brought into extension from the dorsal side by counterpressure. The dorsal pressure distal to the middle joint is applied without touching the splint material (Fig. 4.9b). When modeling,

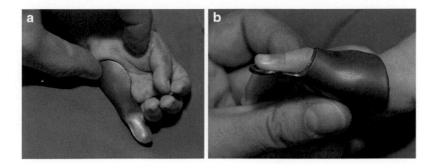

Fig. 4.8 **a** Thermoplastic splint from the palmar side. It covers the palm from the metacarpal bone of the ring finger to the fingertip of the little finger and the edge of the hand to the dorsal side (edges still unprocessed). **b** Splint from the ulnar side. It ends proximal to the middle joint (edges still unprocessed). (© Children's Hospital Wilhelmstift, with kind permission)

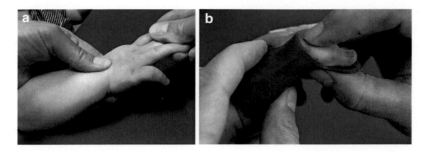

Fig. 4.9 **a** Grasping the wrist and fingers. The wrist is fixed and fingers 2–4 are gently pulled distally so that a little finger splint can be modeled. **b** Modeling a little finger splint. Gently, with one hand, the material is molded around the proximal phalanx and the edge of the hand. The thumb of the other hand pushes the middle joint into extension with the counterpressure of the index finger, which rests proximal to the middle joint. (© Children's Hospital Wilhelmstift, with kind permission)

care must be taken that both the proximal and the distal joint are in a 0° position and are not overextended (Fig. 4.9b). In addition, the little finger must not be pushed into ulnar deviation. It is important to stay close to the ring finger when modeling.

> **Caution:**
> Both the proximal and the distal joint must be encased in the splint in a 0° position. Deviations are prevented by closely aligning with the neighboring finger during modeling.

After modeling, the edges are processed. In the area of the middle finger joint, the splint is minimally "raised" (Chap. 8) to avoid a dorsal

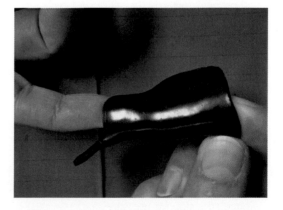

Fig. 4.10 On the dorsal side, the thermoplastic splint is molded dorsally ("raised") at the level of the middle joint, so that no pressure is exerted on it. (© Children's Hospital Wilhelmstift, with kind permission)

pressure point (Fig. 4.10). The splint is marked and mailed to the manufacturer.

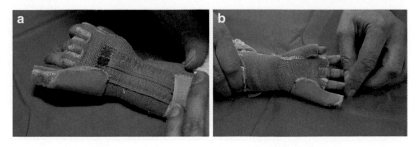

Fig. 4.11 **a** Glove-Splint with integrated thermoplastic splint. **b** The splint is in the pocket and fits snugly against the edge of the hand. The remaining fingers and the wrist are not restricted in their movement by the glove. (© Children's Hospital Wilhelmstift, with kind permission)

Delivery of the Glove-Splint

Approximately two weeks after the order, the glove is completed and delivered.

The handling is explained to the parents as follows:

- The glove is put on without the splint. It must be pulled down deep into the interdigital fold so that the pocket is in the correct position.
- The zipper is closed.
- The splint is now inserted into the small pocket (Fig. 4.5b) and pushed as far distally as possible. It must fit snugly against the edge of the hand (Fig. 4.11a, b). If it sticks out from the edge of the hand, the splint must be shortened towards the palm and back of the hand until it fits optimally.
- The zipper is opened and the glove is pulled back proximally, as the insertion of the splint has shifted the glove distally.
- The splint is now in the correct position, which is checked by palpating the middle joint.
- Due to the distal pocket seam, the glove is slightly longer at the little finger than the specified measurement.
- Before the parents go home with their child, the glove should be worn for about an hour to check the skin for pressure marks.
- If a pressure mark has formed at the middle joint, the position of the splint must be checked again and possibly the "raising" must be reinforced (Fig. 4.10).
- The glove is worn for a few hours during the day for the first 3 to 4 days so that the hand can get used to the compression.

- Parents need to know that due to the compression, the fingers may be a bit colder at the beginning than on the opposite side.
- If the fingers swell, the glove should be slightly pre-stretched.
- After the acclimatization period, the glove is worn for 8 to 12 hours during night sleep.
- The glove must be washed at least once or twice a week at a maximum of 40° Celsius to ensure a tight fit. Fabric softeners and dryers are not allowed as they damage the fabric (washing instructions are always included). The thermoplastic splint must be removed before washing as it is deformed by heat.
- Depending on age, growth spurts and improvement of the contracture, the child needs a new glove and splint every 3 to 8 months.

Glove-Splint
- **Hand position of the holder:**
  Hand 1: Fingers 2–4 are fixed and slightly pulled distally
  Hand 2: The wrist and the distal forearm are fixed
- **Pressure points of the splint:**
  Palmar side= from the palm to the fingertip
  Dorsal side= from the back of the hand to proximal of the middle joint
- **Recommended materials** (Chap. 8):
  – Measurement sheet
  – Tape measure
  – Ruler
  – Pen

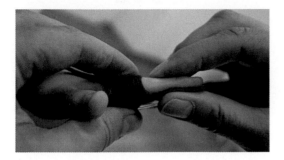

Fig. 4.12 The splint is molded around the index finger, with the two proximal "wings" being spread towards the back of the hand (edges still unprocessed). (© Children's Hospital Wilhelmstift, with kind permission)

- Camera/phone
- Thermoplastic material 2.0 mm, rarely 3.2 mm
- Possibly reins for fixing the splint parts in case of camptodactyly 3&4

Treatment of the Index, Middle, and Ring Fingers

A camptodactyly of the other fingers is much rarer than that of the little finger. However, the therapy is similar. Each finger requires individual adjustment.

Glove-Splint for the Index Finger

The splint for the index finger is molded around the finger similar to the little finger (Fig. 4.12). In the palm and on the back of the hand, the splint continues proximally around the thumb with two small "wings" to ensure sufficient leverage. This does not restrict the movement of the thumb. The opening of the splint pocket is located at the level of the first interdigital fold, crescent-shaped and large enough to guide the splint around the thumb and place it in the pocket (Fig. 4.13a, b).

Glove-Splint for the Middle Finger

For the middle finger, a splint portion is needed from both the palmar and dorsal sides (Fig. 4.14a, b). A strap connects these two parts. Since there is not much space with small fingers, the strap must be sewn as close as possible to the interdigital fold on the glove to fully enclose the dorsal splint portion as well (Fig. 4.14c, d). The thenar muscles and the base joints of the little, ring, and index fingers are not restricted by the splint. The zipper is located on the little finger side.

Glove-Splint for the Ring Finger

A small thermoplastic splint is molded from the palmar tip of the ring finger to the palm and around the edge of the hand. It continues dorsally over the back of the hand to the middle joint of the ring finger. The little finger is completely left out (Fig. 4.15). Since the pressure of the contracture pushes the splint parts apart, this splint, like the splint for the middle finger, needs a strap. The strap holds the splint parts together between the base and middle joint. The base joint of the little finger needs a generous cutout.

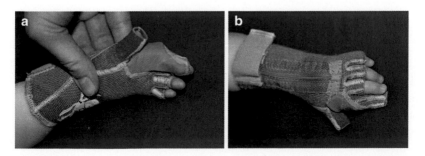

Fig. 4.13 The splint frames the thumb base joint without restricting the thumb's movement. The opening of the pocket is located in the first interdigital fold. (© Children's Hospital Wilhelmstift, with kind permission)

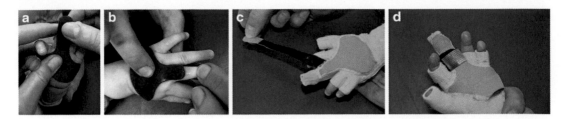

Fig. 4.14 **a** Palmar splint portion for splinting the middle finger (edges still unprocessed). **b** Dorsal splint portion for splinting the middle finger (edges still unprocessed). **c** The strap is attached to the glove fabric between the base and middle joint as close as possible to the interdigital fold. **d** The strap encloses the finger with gentle tension and connects the splint portions. At the pocket opening, the pocket material must still be placed around the end of the splint. This prevents the splint from slipping proximally. (© Children's Hospital Wilhelmstift, with kind permission)

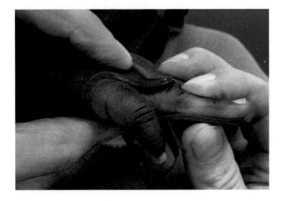

Fig. 4.15 Thermoplastic splint for splinting the ring finger (edges still unprocessed). The splint parts are connected by splint material around the edge of the hand. A not yet existing strap will connect the two splint parts at the level of the finger base phalanxt. (© Children's Hospital Wilhelmstift, with kind permission)

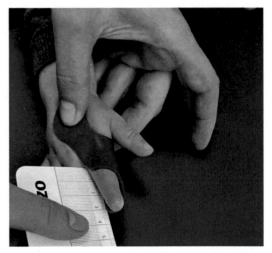

Fig. 4.16 The splint is placed on the finger and the ruler is placed in the interdigital fold. This information serves as a control for the glove manufacturer during the production of the pocket seam. (© Kinderkrankenhaus Wilhelmstift, with kind permission)

Additional Information

- A photo showing both the length of the finger and the respective splint lengths helps the manufacturer to place the pocket in the correct position (Fig. 4.16).
- The rein for connecting the splint parts can only be sewn to the glove fabric, but not to the fabric of the pocket, as otherwise the seam would hinder the insertion of the splint. To fix the finger between the splint parts, the rein must be placed between the base and middle joint or very close to the interdigital fold. A circular encompassing of the finger is important for stability, therefore the material of the rein should be slightly elastic and velcro-attachable, and include velcro at the end. The elasticity of the rein material is of great importance, as the blood circulation of the finger must always be ensured. The rein is included in the delivery. For example, a Buddy loop® is suitable, which is cut to the appropriate length before it is shipped with the splint material (Chap. 8).
- Some children can open the zipper themselves at an early age. To prevent this, a band connects the specially sewn-in hook-eye clasp with the slider (Fig. 4.17).

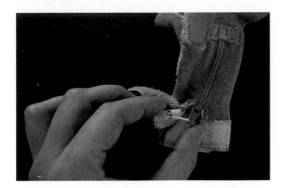

Fig. 4.17 A band between the slider of the zipper and the hook of the hook-eye clasp prevents the child from opening the zipper. (© Kinderkrankenhaus Wilhelmstift, with kind permission)

Caution:
The rein for fixing the splint parts must be made of slightly elastic material so that the blood circulation of the finger is not impaired

4.2.3.2 Dynamic Finger Extension Orthoses

Dynamic finger extension orthoses support the nocturnal splint treatment in cases of severe contractures and late treatment initiation. There are various dynamic finger extension orthoses, also called three-point Quengel splints. Through a spring system, they exert a strong pressure on the middle joint, pushing it into extension (Fig. 4.18b). The pressure points are located on the palmar side on the base joint and proximal to the end joint, on the dorsal side proximal to the

middle joint on the base phalanx. The end joint must not be overstretched by the splint. This splint therapy is performed at least 2 to 3 times a day in intervals of 15 to 30 minutes. If the pressure decreases, the tension of the spring should be increased.

Caution:
The three-point extension splint should only be worn during the day, as the strong pressure can impair circulation after some time.

Some three-point extension splints, with their semi-shell guides of the middle and end piece like those from Ruck MedicalTec© (Chap. 8), have the advantage of guiding the finger out of its rotation position or preventing rotation in the base and middle joint during stretching (Fig. 4.19a–d). To counteract ulnar deviation in the base joint, the little finger can be fixed to the ring finger with a rein, e.g., a Buddy loop® (Fig. 4.19d). The rein on the ring and little finger is located as proximally as possible at the level of the base phalanx. This achieves the best possible stabilization of the little finger base joint radially. If the finger to be treated turns a little redder than the other fingers after a few seconds, the spring pressure is good. If the finger turns blue or white, the pressure must be reduced. The wearing time is gradually increased. The circulation must be checked repeatedly during this time, especially in smaller children.

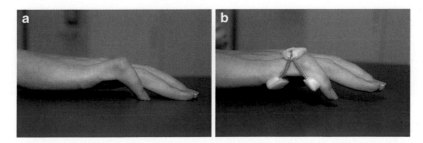

Fig. 4.18 a Severe flexion contracture of the little finger of a 16-year-old with wing-like shortening of the palmar skin. **b** Treatment with a three-point Quengel splint. (© Children's Hospital Wilhelmstift, with kind permission)

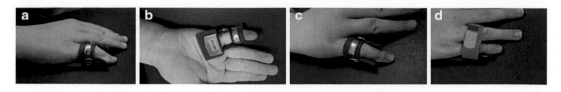

Fig. 4.19 **a** Dynamic finger extension orthosis from Ruck on the hand of a five-year-old. **b** Orthosis from the palmar side. **c** The little finger tends to drift ulnarly in the base joint during stretching. **d** A rein connecting the little finger with the ring finger prevents ulnar deviation. (© Children's Hospital Wilhelmstift, with kind permission)

4.2.3.3 Thermoplastic Static Night Splint

The **thermoplastic static night splint** can replace the Glove-Splint from about the fourth year of life. The night splint is made from 3.2 mm thick thermoplastic, unperforated material. Thinner material is bent by the contracture. The splint is modeled around the finger like the splint for the Glove-Splint. The only difference in shape is that the splint reaches from the palm around the first interdigital fold and ends dorsally approximately at the level of the third metacarpal bone (Fig. 4.20a–d). A rein on the back of the hand and around the base of the little finger connects the parts of the splint. A soft, thin material should be used for the rein on the finger to avoid chafing on the adjacent fingers (Chap. 8). If the splint material has become too thin during modeling or if the force of the flexion contracture is too strong, it can be reinforced with a thermoplastic knitted material, e.g. Orficast® (Fig. 4.20a, b) (Chap. 8). If the distal joint tends to hyperextend, the finger can be fixed in the splint with a rein loop that reaches the fingertip (Fig. 4.20d).

To model the splint, the child is asked to slightly bend the fingers at the base joints to prevent hyperextension of the base joint during the splint production. This way, the joint can be brought into the 0° position in a relaxed hand position. The relaxed hand position also prevents ulnar deviation in the base joint. The little finger is modeled closely to the ring finger. A rein presses the finger into the splint and prevents it from slipping out. If the finger tends to rotate, a soft rein (Chap. 8) at the level of the distal joint can counteract this tendency.

4.2.3.4 Static Night Splint for Positive Tenodesis Tests

A positive tenodesis test indicates a pathological shortening of the extrinsic flexor tendons. In this case, the forearm is included. The wrist is held in the splint at approximately 30° extension to stretch the flexors. The half-shell splint is extended palmarly to the middle of the forearm. Additional straps proximal to the wrist and at the proximal end of the splint secure the splint to the forearm.

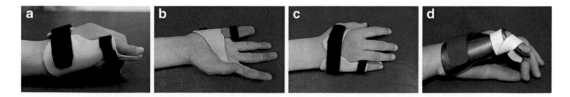

Fig. 4.20 **a** Thermoplastic finger splint with palm enclosure and rein around the little finger. **b** The splint is reinforced palmarly with an additional thermoplastic knitted material to prevent bending due to the force of the contracture. **c** A rein on the little finger fixes it in the splint. **d** With a rein loop, the base phalanx and the distal phalanx are fixed in the splint. This loop is used when the distal joint tends to hyperextend. (© Children's Hospital Wilhelmstift, with kind permission)

Thermoplastic Static Night Splint
- **Hand position of the holder:**
  Hand 1: Fingers 2 to 4 are fixed and slightly pulled distally.
  Hand 2: the wrist and the distal forearm are fixed.
- **Pressure points of the palm splint:**
  Palmar = from the palm to the fingertip
  Dorsal = from the back of the hand to proximal of the finger middle joint
  Radial = first interdigital fold
  Ulnar = edge of the hand to the little finger middle joint

Static Night Splint for Positive Tenodesis Test
- **Hand position of the holder:**
  Hand 1: Fingers 2 to 4 are fixed and slightly pulled distally
  Hand 2: the proximal forearm is fixed
- **Pressure points of the palm splint:**
  Palmar = from the forearm to the fingertip
  Dorsal = from the back of the hand to proximal of the finger middle joint, additionally via Velcro fasteners on the

back of the hand, proximal of the wrist and at the proximal end of the splint
Radial and ulnar = a half-shell shape prevents the hand from deviating radially or ulnarly
- **Recommended materials** (Chap. 8):
  - Thermoplastic material 3.2 mm
  - Composite material to reinforce the splint on the palmar side (e.g. Orficast)
  - Fleece tape
  - Velcro fastener

4.2.3.5 Orthotic Therapy

If flexion contractures occur on several fingers (Fig. 4.21a), in addition to intensive manual treatment, **orthotic therapy** is used.

Manual treatment is performed on all affected fingers. It is extremely important for the success of the treatment, as only through manual therapy the maximum extension of the middle joints can be achieved. In older children, exercises to strengthen the extrinsic and intrinsic muscles are actively adopted. The focus is on practicing selective extension in the middle joint while blocking the base joint and on the lumbrical grip (Sec. 4.2.4). If there are axis deviations, exercises for abduction or adduction in the base joints are necessary depending on the findings.

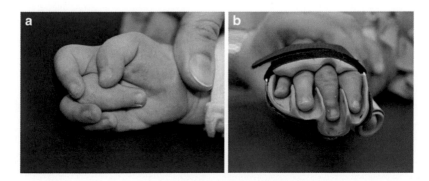

Fig. 4.21 **a** 10-month-old girl with flexion contractures of all fingers, the flexion contracture of the middle finger middle joint is most pronounced. **b** Orthosis for the treatment of multiple finger flexion contractures. The different finger contractures are compensated for from the palmar side, the thickened middle joint of the middle finger additionally receives a generous cutout in the dorsal pad. The fingers are also supported laterally to counteract deviation. This is not yet fully possible with the index finger. After a wearing time of 20 min, the middle finger became livid. By gently grinding away the splint material, the contracture was slightly accommodated, so that the circulation was sufficiently improved. (© Children's Hospital Wilhelmstift, with kind permission)

Nighttime orthosis therapy also supports manual therapy here. Due to the individual finger enclosure required for the correct fit, the skills and technical capabilities of an orthopedic technician are needed to manufacture such an orthosis. The forearm orthosis with individual finger enclosure always includes all three-jointed fingers, even if a finger is not affected, as the pulleys of the finger pad need space radially and ulnarly (Fig. 4.21b). The orthosis is made from Streifi-Flex and/or carbon and encompasses the forearm and the hand shell-like from the palmar side. Different degrees of finger flexion contractures are compensated from the palmar side. The dorsal pad pushes the fingers into the orthosis at the level of the finger base phalanges. The pad only compensates for small height differences of the finger base phalanges. Inter-finger guides prevent skin-to-skin contact and the fingers from slipping to the side. The finger base and end joints must not be overstretched. They remain in extension or a slight flexion of 10°. The finger middle joints are stretched as far as possible, but painlessly, in the orthosis. The proximal part of the orthosis covers about 2/3 of the forearm length to achieve a sufficient lever. The dorsal straps are located at the finger base phalanges, proximal to the wrist, and at the proximal end of the orthosis. Sometimes a strap over the back of the hand is needed. The orthosis is made after a plaster cast or 3D scan (Chap. 8).

Forearm orthosis with individual finger enclosure

- **Hand and finger position in the orthosis:**
  Wrist—Extension to dorsal side (up to a maximum of 30° extension).
  Fingers 2 to 5—maximum stretching of the middle joints. The base and end joints remain in 0° to 10° flexion in individual finger enclosure with finger bridges.
  Thumb is enclosed in functional position, or in gentle abduction.
- **Orthosis enclosure:**
  Approximately 2/3 of the circumference of the forearm and hand are enclosed from the palmar side.
  About 2/3 of the length of the forearm is enclosed, the hand completely.
- **Pressure points:**
  Palmar side: from the forearm to the fingertip. Different finger contractures are compensated from the palmar side over the orthosis
  Dorsal side: Strap at the level of the distal forearm close to the wrist, attachment on the proximal forearm, finger pad between base and middle joints/at the level of the distal base phlanges
- **Recommended materials** (Chap. 8):
  – Streifi-Flex
  – Carbon brace
  – Deflector
  – Strap with Velcro fastener
  – Finger pad

Caution:
No deviation and hyperextension in the base joints. Different finger flexion contractures must be compensated for in the orthosis over the palmar side. The dorsal finger pad can only compensate for small differences.

4.2.4 Advanced manual therapy

Since muscular imbalances are largely involved in the malposition of the middle joint, active exercises should supplement passive stretching. From primary school age, the exercises can be trained with the child.

In most children and adolescents, during the active extension of the affected finger

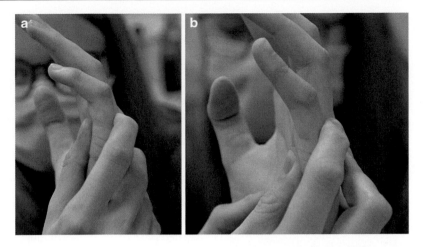

Fig. 4.22 **a** Fixing the base joint to avoid hyperextension. **b** Active extension in the middle joint against the resistance of the holding hand. (© Kinderkrankenhaus Wilhelmstift, with kind permission)

- a hyperextension in the base joint,
- a deviation to the ulnar side,
- a rotation towards the thumb,

is usually observed in combination.

If this is the case, not only the extensors should be actively stretched to improve mobility of the PIP joint, but also the interosseous and lumbrical muscles.

In older children and adolescents, the tenodesis test is performed before starting the exercises. If it is positive, the wrist should be held in extension during therapy, as this maximally stretches the flexor tendons.

Therapy suggestions for advanced manual therapy:

4.2.4.1 Exercises for the extrinsic muscles

- The patient fixes the base joint with the unaffected hand in a 0° position and actively extends the affected finger in the middle joint (Fig. 4.22a, b). It must be ensured that the little finger is close to the ring finger. The finger is held in extension for 10 to 20 seconds. These exercises should be performed 4–5 times a day with 30 repetitions each.

4.2.4.2 Exercises for the intrinsic muscles

- The finger is placed in the lumbrical position (Chap. 1). This means that the base joints are

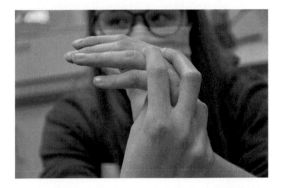

Fig. 4.23 The base joints are held in a flexed position. The middle joint is actively extended and pressed against the holding hand. (© Kinderkrankenhaus Wilhelmstift, with kind permission)

held in flexion and the middle and end joints are actively extended (Fig. 4.23). It must be ensured that the little finger does not deviate ulnarly, but lies against the ring finger. Additionally, pressure can be applied to the base phalanx with the unaffected hand to intensify the extension in the middle joint.

- A sponge is placed between the ring and little finger, the little finger tries to press the sponge against the ring finger. The base joints are in flexion to avoid hyperextension and direct the strengthening directly to the intrinsic muscles.

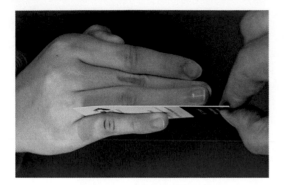

Fig. 4.24 The base joints are in flexion, the middle and end joints in extension. The little finger presses the business card against the ring finger and forcefully prevents the card from being pulled out. (© Kinderkrankenhaus Wilhelmstift, with kind permission)

- A business card is placed between the ring and little finger. The little finger presses it forcefully against the ring finger. With the unaffected hand, an attempt is now made to pull out the business card (Fig. 4.24). A slight flexion in the base joints is important to avoid hyperextension and to specifically strengthen the intrinsic muscles.

4.2.4.3 Training the central slip

To concentrate the stretching exercises on the central slip and block the lateral bands (Fig. 4.25a), an Oval-8 splint can be made. This holds the end joint at 0° (Fig. 4.25b). Also with this stretching exercise, the base joint may need

to be blocked by the unaffected hand to avoid hyperextension. With practice the patient should actively practice preventing hyperextension during extension on his own.

▶ The exercises or positions are each held for 20 to 30 seconds, repeated 30 times, and performed 4–5 times a day. The more frequently the exercises are performed, the better the results.

4.2.5　Postoperative treatment

If surgery is required despite intensive conservative treatment, postoperative treatment is carried out after wound closure or after removal of a joint-fixing Kirschner wire.

4.2.5.1 Case Study

A nearly 16-year-old patient presents herself. The proximal interphalangeal joint of the right hand's little finger is spontaneously in 90° flexion (Fig. 4.26), the fist closure is complete. Due to the therapy-resistant camptodactyly, surgery is performed (Fig. 4.27a, b).

Surgery: After the transverse incision, the neurovascular bundles are exposed. The nerves and arteries are taut like a bowstring. The ulnar transposition flap is mobilized, the flexor tendon sheath between the A2 and A3 annular ligament is opened transversely, the superficial flexor

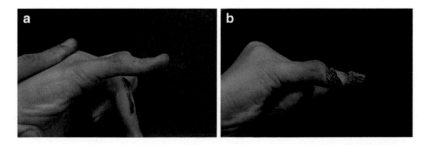

Fig. 4.25 **a** 12-year-old girl with camptodactyly. The middle joint was stretched by intensive splint treatment. There is a clear hyperextension in the end joint with almost complete middle joint extension. **b** The hyperextension was prevented by an Oval-8 ring. The extension of the little finger is now much more difficult for the patient. The focus of the training is the active extension in the middle joint. Since the splint exerts a considerable pressure on the dorsal middle phalanx during extension, this splint is only an exercise splint. (© Kinderkrankenhaus Wilhelmstift, with kind permission)

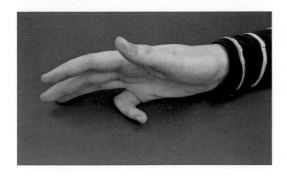

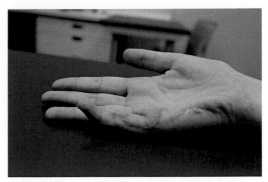

Fig. 4.26 16-year-old patient with therapy-resistant camptodactyly. The proximal interphalangeal joint of the little finger is spontaneously in 90° flexion, it can be passively extended to 70° with a lot of force. Active extension beyond 90° is not possible. (© Kinderkrankenhaus Wilhelmstift, with kind permission)

Fig. 4.28 Same patient, fourth postoperative week. The K-wire has been removed. The scar is red and immature. Start of splint therapy and manual treatment. (© Kinderkrankenhaus Wilhelmstift, with kind permission)

tendon is severed. This is followed by arthrolysis with severing of the palmar plate, the arthrolysis is carried out until the middle joint can be freely extended. Due to the reduced blood flow in the extended position, caused by the strong pull on the short palmar blood vessels, the middle joint is set in 40° flexion and fixed with a K-wire. The ulnar transposition flap is placed over the middle joint, the remaining skin defects are covered with skin grafts.

The **manual treatment and splint therapy** begins after the cast and the K-wire are removed, starting from the fourth postoperative week (Fig. 4.28).

It should be carried out for at least four months, as the scar tension is strongest during the remodeling processes in this period (Chap. 6). Post-treatment during the entire scar maturation period, i.e., for one year, is recommended.

It focuses on:

- the movement into flexion and extension,
- the strengthening of the intrinsic and extrinsic musculature,
- the scar treatment,
- the prevention of a recurrence.

Both manual and splint treatment are almost identical to the preoperative treatment and are supplemented by scar massage (Chap. 6), silicone treatment (Chap. 6) and exercise splints.

4.2.5.2 Glove-Splint, Silicone Gel
The static splint treatment for contracture prophylaxis and scar treatment can also be carried out

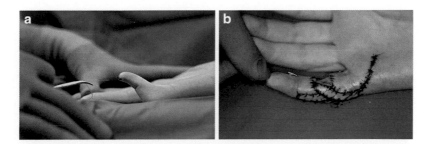

Fig. 4.27 **a** Preparation of the finger for surgery. A thread has already been passed through the fingertip and the end of the nail for fixation. **b** At the end of the surgery. The middle joint is in 40° flexion and is fixed with a K-wire, the ulnar transposition flap has been placed over the middle joint and the remaining skin defects have been covered with skin grafts. (© Kinderkrankenhaus Wilhelmstift, with kind permission)

in older patients using a **glove-splint**. To use the glove-splint for scar treatment, the circumference of the finger and the palm must be measured with a slight pull (Fig. 4.6b). This achieves sufficient compression. The inserted splint keeps the finger in the desired extension and counteracts the scar pull and the forming of a new contracture.

If additional silicone treatment is desired, it can only be carried out simultaneously with a glove-splint using **silicone gel** or a second compression stocking with Silon-Tex. Sewn-in Silon-Tex (Chap. 6) is not possible in the glove-splint, as Silon-Tex cannot be applied from the inside and the splint pocket from the outside at the same time. More effective than the silicone gel is a second compression stocking with Silon-Tex, which is worn alternately with the glove-splint.

4.2.5.3 Compression Stocking with Silon-Tex, Thermoplastic Splint

As a variant, a **compression stocking with Silon-Tex** (Chap. 6) and a **thermoplastic splint** attached over the glove can be used (Fig. 4.38a–c). After removal of the K-wire, the finger must be splinted for about 16 hours daily for four months. Afterwards, the wearing time can be reduced to the duration of the night's sleep and the silicone can be omitted depending on the condition of the scar.

After removal of the K-wire, manual therapy (Sect. 4.2.4) must be carried out intensively at least 4–5 times a day for four months in order to achieve good mobility and strengthening of the finger.

4.2.5.4 Dynamic Flexion Splint

To support manual treatment, splints can be made for practicing both flexion (Fig. 4.29a, b) and extension (Fig. 4.30a, b). This **dynamic flexion splint** fixes the base joint and pulls the middle joint into flexion. The rein can regulate the force of the flexion.

4.2.5.5 Relative-Motion-Splint

A **Relative-Motion-Splint** can be made for active extension exercises of the middle joint (Fig. 4.30a, b). By blocking the little finger base joint, its hyperextension is prevented. From this position, the little finger middle joint is actively brought into extension. Six months postoperatively, the middle joint can be actively extended up to 20° and flexed up to 70° (Fig. 4.31a, b).

4.2.6 Treatment Examples

4.2.6.1 Camptodactyly of the Middle Finger

This infant was presented to us at the age of 5 months. The little boy shows a camptodactyly of the middle finger. The middle joint could only be extended to 90° passively. With passive extension, a strong flexor tendon pull from the middle joint to the palm was noticeable (Fig. 4.32a).

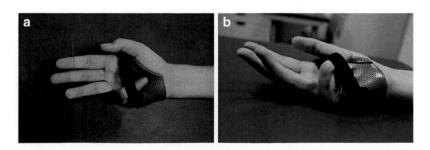

Fig. 4.29 a, b Dynamic flexion splint for practicing the flexion of the middle joint. The rein regulates the force of the flexion. (© Children's Hospital Wilhelmstift, with kind permission)

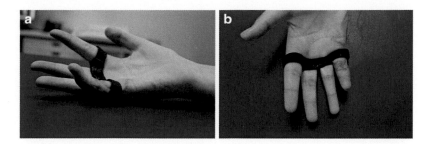

Fig. 4.30 a Relative-Motion-Splint for active extension exercises of the middle joint. From the slight flexion position of the little finger base joint, the finger is actively brought into extension. The block dorso-proximal of the middle joint leads to a better active extension of the joint. **b** The Relative-Motion-Splint prevents the hyperextension of the little finger base joint during the extension exercises. (© Children's Hospital Wilhelmstift, with kind permission)

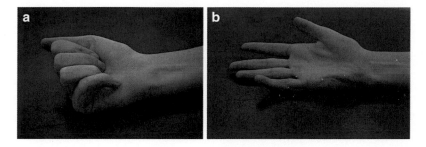

Fig. 4.31 a, b Same patient. Check-up 6 months postoperatively, The middle joint can be actively extended to 20° and flexed to 70°. Passive extension is possible up to 0° and flexion up to 80°. (© Children's Hospital Wilhelmstift, with kind permission)

Initially, intensive manual treatment by physiotherapists and parents was started. From the 10th month of life, the little boy received Glove-Splints for nightly extension of the middle finger for a year.

After this year, only manual therapy was continued with a remaining passive extension deficit of 20° (Fig. 4.32b).

At the age of four years, the boy needed a thermoplastic splint for the night due to a deterioration during a growth spurt.

After a 6-month treatment, an active extension deficit of 20° remained, passively the finger was fully extendable (Fig. 4.33). The manual treatment was carried out twice a day during all this time.

4.2.6.2 Camptodactyly of the Little Finger

At the age of 22 months, we saw this boy with a camptodactyly of the right little finger (Fig. 4.34a).

Passively, the finger could only be extended to 80° in the middle joint. Manual therapy began on the same day, and treatment with the Glove-Splint started two weeks later.

After 9 months of treatment, a passive extension deficit of 30° remained (Fig. 4.34b). The splint treatment was continued for a year, and the manual treatment was continued until primary school age (Fig. 4.34c). At the age of 7 years, the finger could be fully extended actively.

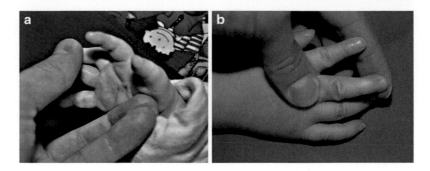

Fig. 4.32 a 5-month-old boy with camptodactyly of the middle finger. The middle joint can only be extended passively up to 90°. The shortened palmar skin is clearly tense up to the palm. **b** At the age of 2 years, after intensive manual therapy and splint treatment, there is only a remaining extension deficit of 20°. (© Children's Hospital Wilhelmstift, with kind permission)

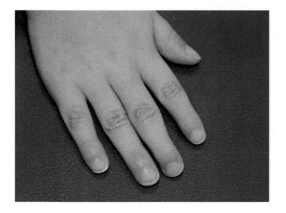

Fig. 4.33 At the age of almost 5 years. Due to a deterioration during a growth spurt, the manual therapy was supported by a night splint for 6 months at the age of four years. The finger could then be actively extended to 20°. Passive full extension was possible with pressure. (© Children's Hospital Wilhelmstift, with kind permission)

▶ **Success can only be achieved and maintained with consistent manual stretching and active exercise treatment**

4.2.6.3 Multiple Flexion Contractures

This girl was presented at the age of 10 months. The right hand showed flexion contractures of fingers 2 to 5. The middle finger was completely folded into the palm. The middle joint could not be extended even passively. A deficit of 100° remained in extension (Fig. 4.35a).

The index finger showed, in addition to the flexion contracture in the middle joint, an ulnar deviation at the level of the base joint. The palm could not be fully widened passively.

Manual treatment began on the same day. The orthosis was made three weeks later, after

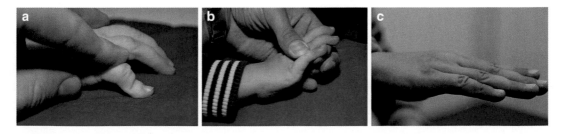

Fig. 4.34 a 22-month-old boy with a passive extension deficit in the middle joint of 80° with a hard stop. **b** The contracture of the middle joint could be reduced to a passive extension deficit of 30° after consistent treatment over 9 months. **c** At the age of 7 years, the little finger's middle joint is fully extendable both actively and passively. (© Children's Hospital Wilhelmstift, with kind permission)

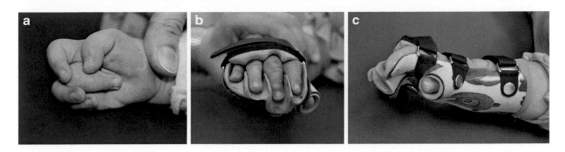

Fig. 4.35 a 10-month-old girl with flexion contractures of all fingers, most pronounced at the middle joint of the middle finger. **b** The different finger contractures are compensated from the palmar side, the thickened middle joint of the middle finger additionally receives a cutout in the dorsal pad. The fingers are also supported laterally to counteract deviation. After a wearing time of 20 min, the middle finger became livid. By gently grinding away the splint material, the contracture was slightly accommodated and blood circulation sufficiently improved. **c** The thumb is included in the splint to widen the palm. The wrist is in 30° extension to stretch the flexors. (© Children's Hospital Wilhelmstift, with kind permission)

manual therapy had already slightly improved the contractures.

In the orthosis, fingers 2 to 5 were splinted using individual finger enclosures and the different contractures of the fingers were compensated from the palmar side. The thickened middle joint of the middle finger required a generous cutout in the dorsal pad (Fig. 4.35b). The ulnar deviation of the index finger was slightly counteracted by the tall finger guidance from the ulnar and radial sides.

The thumb received a casing to fully widen the palm also in width (Fig. 4.35b, c). The wrist was placed in 30° extension to stretch the flexors (Fig. 4.35c).

After 4 months of treatment, the girl needed a new splint due to reduced contractures and an increase in hand size. At this time, the palm could be fully extended passively and all fingers could be better extended actively (Fig. 4.36a, b). Passively, all fingers except the middle finger could be fully extended with force (Fig. 4.36b). The hand was used much better actively. Spontaneously, the index, ring, and little fingers were still slightly flexed. During bimanual gripping, the middle finger interfered due to its remaining flexed position. To intensify the extension of the middle finger middle joint, the treatment was supplemented by a dynamic finger extension orthosis during the day. In the case of this little girl, the finger extension orthosis could

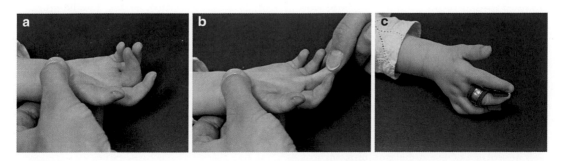

Fig. 4.36 a Spontaneously, the middle finger is in 90° flexion. **b** All middle joints except that of the middle finger can be fully extended passively. The middle finger can be extended passively up to 70°. There is a clear pull visible from the palm to the tip of the middle finger. **c** A dynamic finger extension orthosis supports manual treatment during the day. It can only be worn for 10 min at a time, as the blood circulation (despite the light setting of the spring) quickly decreases. (© Children's Hospital Wilhelmstift, with kind permission)

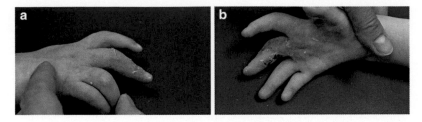

Fig. 4.37 **a** Spontaneously, the middle finger is in 40° flexion. **b** 8 weeks postoperatively. There are still crusts on the palmar side of the middle finger. (© Children's Hospital Wilhelmstift, with kind permission)

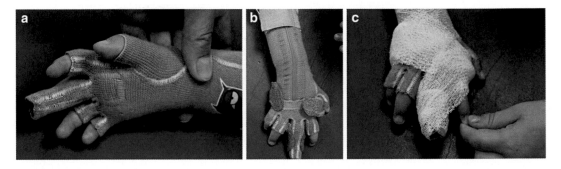

Fig. 4.38 **a** A compression glove with sewn-in Silon-Tec treats the scars. **b** A small thermoplastic splint made of Orficast® splints the finger in extension. **c** The splint is fixed to the hand with Peha-haft®, the slight pull to the radial side is intended to counteract the ulnar deviation in the base joint. This supply is worn for about 12 hours during night sleep. (© Children's Hospital Wilhelmstift, with kind permission)

only be worn for 10 min at a time, as the blood circulation deteriorated after a short time despite the only slight tension of the spring (Fig. 4.36c) (Chap. 8).

After 14 months of consistent conservative treatment, all fingers except the middle finger are freely extendable. The middle finger remains in a flexion contracture of 90° and a maximum extension of 50° with a very firm stop in the middle joint and strong pull of the skin and flexor tendon. The palmar space between the base and end joint has hardly increased. At the age of two, the middle finger is surgically corrected (Fig. 4.37a, b).

An arthrolysis is performed with opening of the flexor tendon sheath, a tenolysis of the superficial and deep flexor tendon, an arterio- and neurolysis of the radial and ulnar neurovascular bundles, the opening of the palmar plate, and a partial detachment of the M. lumbricalis. The complex operation is followed by intensive post-treatment.

Due to the delayed wound healing, compression treatment with Silon-Tec for scar treatment can only be started 10 weeks postoperatively (Fig. 4.38a–c) (Chap. 6). Over the glove, a small thermoplastic splint is worn, which keeps the finger in the best possible extension, (Fig. 4.38b, c) and is attached to the glove with Peha-haft® (Fig. 4.38c) (Chap. 8). Due to the slight ulnar deviation of the middle finger in the base joint, it is braced radially by the Peha-haft®. The glove and splint are worn for about 12 hours during night sleep, during the day the hand remains free for exercise and play. The child receives physiotherapy.

References

Guy Foucher MD (2006) 6 Boulevard Edwards Strasbourg, France 67000 IFSSH@aol.com

David TN MD (2015) 6624 Fannin Street, Suite 2730 Houston Texas 7730, netscher@bcm.dedu

Arthrogryposis

5

Contents

5.1 Symptom Picture

Arthrogryposis is not a specific diagnosis, but a **symptom complex** found in more than 300 disease patterns. This disease pattern is characterized by congenital, non-progressive (= advancing) restrictions of joint mobility up to joint stiffness due to missing, altered and/or underdeveloped musculature. The affected muscles are replaced by connective or adipose tissue (Mundlos and Horn 2014). Active movements, which are necessary for joint formation, cannot be performed. The children are born with malpositions of the shoulders, arms and hands, and often also of the hips, legs and feet (Fig. 5.1) (Bahm 2017). The restrictions and malpositions vary greatly and range from a thumb-in-palm deformity to malposition of numerous joints. Organ damage is also possible. Sensory innervation and body perception are undisturbed, the central feedback is intact, but the motor implementation is disturbed (Bahm 2017).

In order to better assess the extent of functional restrictions, arthrogryposis is classified as follows:

- classic arthrogryposis multiplex congenita (AMC),
- distal arthrogryposis,
- syndromal arthrogryposis.

Arthros	Joint
Gryposis	Curved
Multiplex	Multiple
Congenital	Hereditary

Different classifications of AMC can be found in the literature, the following two capture the severity from different perspectives:

Classification of the AMC Interest Group
→ focuses on the **restrictions in everyday life**.

- Type 1: Only the extremities are affected. This group is divided into two degrees of severity:
  1. Changes to the hands and feet without involvement of the proximal joints.
  2. Changes to the entire extremities including elbow, knee, shoulder and hip joints.

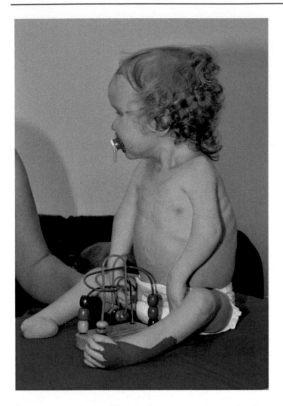

Fig. 5.1 15-month-old girl with a severe form of arthrogryposis multiplex congenita. (© Children's Hospital Wilhelmstift, with kind permission)

- Type 2: Changes as in type 1 plus organ malformations such as of the abdominal wall/ gastroschisis
- Type 3: Joint stiffness plus malformations of the spine and the central or peripheral nervous system.

Classification According to Affected Segment Level
→ is oriented towards the **severity levels of anatomical restrictions**.

The classification by Brown 1980, which was modified by Agranovich and Lakhinal 2020, is based on the level of the affected spinal cord segment/ myotome.

Two main forms are distinguished:

- the complex form
- the isolated form.

In the complex form, AMC is combined with other pathologies, such as cerebral disorders.

The isolated form is divided into four types, corresponding to the classification of segmental injuries to the cervical and lumbar vertebral bodies (Tbl. 5.1) (Agranovich and Lakhinal 2020):

Type 1:		
[-C6-C7-]		
Shoulder	passive	functional
	active	functional or slightly restricted
Elbow	passive	functional or slightly restricted
	active	Active flexion is limited or not possible, active supination is limited
Wrist	passive	functional or slightly restricted
	active	Active flexion is maintained, active extension is limited or not possible
Finger & Thumb	passive & active	Functional or slightly restricted, some patients exhibit finger contractures and possibly restricted abduction of the thumb

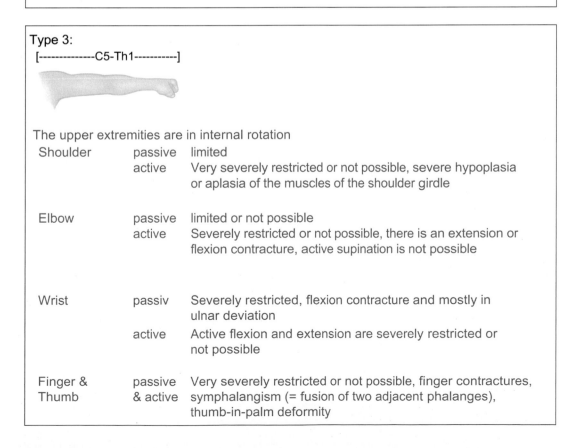

Type 2:
  [---------C5-C7--------]

Shoulder	passive active	Functional oder moderately restricted- restricted - Abduction 30-45° - musculature of the shoulder girdle is hypoplastic
Elbow	passive active	functional or moderately restricted Active flexion is severely restricted or not possible, active supination is not possible
Wrist	passive active	severely restricted, Flexion contracture with ulnar deviation Active flexion is restricted, active extension is restricted or not possible
Finger & Thumb	passive & active	Mild or moderate restrictions, some patients exhibit finger contractures, possible thumb-in-palm deformity

Type 3:
  [-------------C5-Th1----------]

The upper extremities are in internal rotation

Shoulder	passive active	limited Very severely restricted or not possible, severe hypoplasia or aplasia of the muscles of the shoulder girdle
Elbow	passive active	limited or not possible Severely restricted or not possible, there is an extension or flexion contracture, active supination is not possible
Wrist	passiv active	Severely restricted, flexion contracture and mostly in ulnar deviation Active flexion and extension are severely restricted or not possible
Finger & Thumb	passive & active	Very severely restricted or not possible, finger contractures, symphalangism (= fusion of two adjacent phalanges), thumb-in-palm deformity

Type 4:

C6
|

Shoulder	passive	functional
	active	Functional or slightly restricted, muscles of the shoulder girdle only slightly hypoplastic
Elbow	passive	Functional to severely restricted
	active	Full extension possible, flexion is slightly to severely restricted
Wrist	passive	functional or limited,
	active	
Finger & Thumb	passive	Good function
	active	

▶ **Myotomes** are muscular primordial segments of the embryo.

Misalignments and Movement Restrictions of the Upper Extremities

In severe forms of AMC, the muscles of the shoulders, arms, and hands, as well as in many cases also the hips, legs, and feet, are hypotrophic or atrophied, and the joints show flexion or extension contractures. The children have very different restrictions and misalignments. The following overview describes movement restrictions of the joints of the upper extremities from proximal to distal.

5.1.1 Shoulder Joints

The shoulder joints can be unaffected to severely affected. In severe cases, there is adduction and internal rotation (Fig. 5.2a). Due to the limited active mobility, the range of motion of the arms is greatly restricted. Even passively, mobility is limited (Fig. 5.2c). The

muscles are hypotrophic. The arms are swung into the desired position using gravity and trunk movement (Fig. 5.2b).

5.1.2 Elbows

The elbows can be actively freely mobile, have limited mobility, or exhibit a complete loss of movement. The forearms can be pronated (Fig. 5.2a–c), with active supination not possible and passive supination incomplete. The children help themselves by hyperextending their backs and applying counterpressure with their hands on a solid surface to bring their shoulders into anteversion and thereby keep their elbows extended. In this position, for example a pencil can be guided to write or paint (Fig. 5.3a). The range of motion is limited to a very small space. If the elbow joints can be passively flexed, a table edge can be used to establish hand-mouth contact. Usually, the other arm serves as a support or counterpressure for the executing arm (Fig. 5.3b).

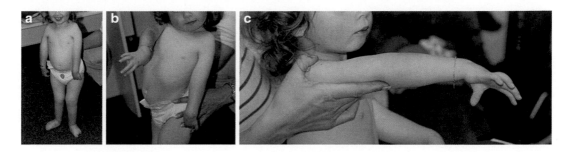

Fig. 5.2 a. 2-year-old girl, the shoulder joints are in adduction and internal rotation. The muscles are weak. **b** The elbow joints can be flexed passively, but not actively. The forearms are in pronation, the wrists in flexion. By changing the center of gravity and swinging the upper body, the arms are passively brought into another position. **c** Even the passive mobility of the shoulder joints is limited. The thumbs are tucked in at the hand (thumb-in-palm deformity). The middle joints of fingers 2–5 are flexed, the base joints tend to hyperextend in compensation with little active extension. (© Children's Hospital Wilhelmstift, with kind permission)

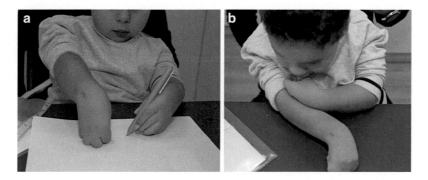

Fig. 5.3 a 5-year-old boy with AMC. Counterpressure between the body and table extends the right elbow joint, stabilizing the upper body while the left hand paints. **b** Passive elbow flexion is achieved by pressing the upper body onto the left arm against the table, establishing hand-mouth contact. The upper body leans towards the hand, the right arm is used as counterpressure. (© Kinderkrankenhaus Wilhelmstift, with kind permission)

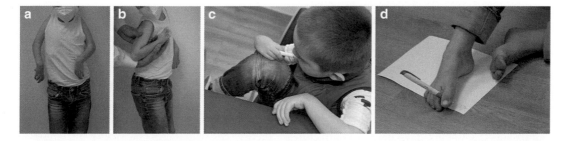

Fig. 5.4 a–b 7-year-old boy with elbow flexion contracture due to severe AMC of the upper extremities. **b** The elbow joints can be passively flexed. **c** The right leg is used to bring the hand to the mouth. **d** He writes with his skilled feet. (© Kinderkrankenhaus Wilhelmstift, with kind permission)

5.1.2.1 Flexion Contracture

Much less common is a **flexion contracture** of the elbow with passive mobility in flexion (Fig. 5.4a–c). Active movement is severely limited or not possible, the arms are pronated. In the case of an existing flexion contracture of the elbow, care must be taken during the child's development that the contracture does not

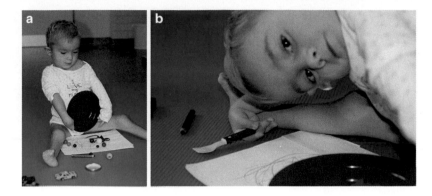

Fig. 5.5 **a** 3-year-old boy with severe AMC. The shoulder girdle is hypoplastic, the forearms are in pronation, the elbows have extension contractures, the hand and finger joints have flexion contractures. The muscles of the upper and lower extremities are hypotrophic or atrophied. **b** Extension contractures of the elbows do not allow hand-mouth contact. (© Kinderkrankenhaus Wilhelmstift, with kind permission)

worsen and thereby further restricts the range of motion. If the condition worsens, orthotic therapy may be indicated in addition to manual treatment.

If the lower extremities are well mobile, the legs can flex the elbows and thus enable hand-mouth contact (Fig. 5.4c). With good mobility and skilled feet, these take over hand functions, such as writing and brushing teeth (Fig. 5.4d). Often, however, the lower extremities are also severely affected, so this compensation is not possible (Fig. 5.1).

5.1.2.2 Extension Contracture

In the most severe form, there is an **extension contracture** of the elbows. These can then also not be moved passively. In addition, there is a serious hypoplasia or aplasia of the shoulder girdle muscles. Usually, movements can only be transferred from the trunk to the arms by the child. The forearms are in pronation, the wrists are flexed, the thumbs are tucked into the palm, and the fingers have flexion contractures (Fig. 5.5a). This malposition does not allow hand-mouth contact (Fig. 5.5b). Independent eating is very difficult and only possible with a bent upper body and a tool, e.g., an extended fork or spoon. The children are completely dependent on outside help and/or aids. Surgical interventions followed by weeks of intensive manual therapy and splint treatment are

unavoidable in order to give the child a greater degree of independence by achieving passive elbow mobility.

▶ **Overview**

An elbow extension contracture does not allow hand-mouth contact.

Passive mobility of the elbow is of great importance for the child's independence.

5.1.3 Wrists

5.1.3.1 Flexion Contracture

The wrists are often in a **flexion contracture** (Fig. 5.6a–c). Active flexion is severely limited, active extension is hardly possible. Even passively, the wrists are not extendable from infancy (Fig. 5.6b).

If toddlers with AMC cannot walk, they move by sliding on their buttocks. They support themselves with the dorsal side of the contracted wrists (Fig. 5.6c). This worsens the flexion deformity of the wrists. If sliding on the buttocks is the only active means of locomotion for the child, it should not be inhibited.

To achieve the largest possible range of motion of the wrists, daily manual treatment is supported with nightly splint therapy from infancy. Depending on the severity, the wrist

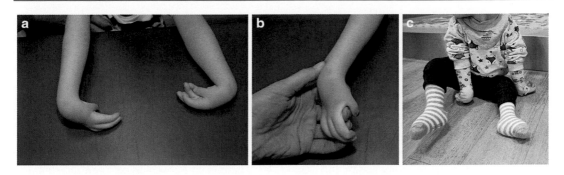

Fig. 5.6 a 3-year-old boy with extension contracture of the elbows, pronation position of the forearms, flexion contractures of the wrists and fingers, and a thumb-in-palm deformity. **b** The wrists can only be slightly flexed even passively. **c** 1.5-year-old boy with a severe form of AMC. The boy moves by sliding his buttocks, supporting himself on the backs of his hands. (© Children's Hospital Wilhelmstift, with kind permission)

position can be significantly improved through conservative therapy. Even if surgery is indicated, splint therapy should pre-stretch the wrist as much as possible beforehand.

5.1.3.2 Extension Contracture

Children with a syndromal arthrogryposis such as Freeman-Sheldon or Sheldon-Hall syndrome often have **extension contractures** of the wrists. Flexion is limited. This extension contracture is not as severe as the flexion contracture. However, movement to at least 0° is useful to facilitate smooth movements, such as putting on and taking off clothes, brushing teeth, drying off, combing, writing. A larger range of motion of the wrists requires fewer compensatory movements of the elbows and shoulders, thus reducing the high strain.

▶ Missing motion creases indicate passively and actively restricted joints.

5.1.4 Fingers, Thumb and Metacarpus

The entire hand, metacarpus, thumb and finger joints are often flexed (Fig. 5.7a). When attempting to extend the fingers, the base joints of fingers 2–5 and the thumb end joints are often hyperextended (compensatory hyperextension position), while the other joints remain in flexion (Fig. 5.2c). In severe cases, the intrinsic hand muscles are weak and not very functional, and the extrinsic muscles are nonfunctional. Wrist contractures further reduce the strength and range of motion of the fingers. Due to the shortening of the palmar soft

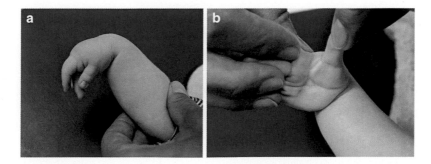

Fig. 5.7 a 4-month-old girl. The wrist is spontaneously in 70° flexion, the thumb points towards the palm, the fingers are flexed. **b** When passively straightening the wrist, thumb and fingers, a palmar tension of the soft tissues becomes visible both in the area of the thumb base joint as well as the palm. (© Children's Hospital Wilhelmstift, with kind permission)

tissues, the palm cannot be fully opened even passively (Fig. 5.7b). Fingers 2–5 cannot be brought into flexion and extension completely or at all, and the fist cannot be closed actively or passively.

5.1.4.1 Passive Hyperextension of the Finger Joints

Some finger joints can be unstable in addition to being contracted. In many cases, the instability manifests as a **passive hyperextension of the finger joints**. This primarily affects the metacarpophalangeal and proximal interphalangeal joints of fingers 2–5 and the distal joint of the thumb. Dimples on the dorsal side over the proximal interphalangeal joints and the thumb's distal joint are signs of an unstable volar plate (Fig. 5.8a, b) (Chap. 1). To prevent deterioration, hyperextensions must be avoided during therapy. These joints are encased in a splint in a slight flexion of approximately 20°.

5.1.4.2 Windblown hand deformity

In addition, fingers 2–5 can exhibit a so-called **windblown hand deformity** (Fig. 5.9a–c), i.e., an ulnar malposition of the fingers at the metacarpophalangeal joints (Chap. 1). This malposition reduces the strength of the fingers and makes opposition weaker, more imprecise, and in combination with a severe thumb-in-palm deformity, impossible.

5.1.4.3 Thumb-in-Palm Deformity

In severe forms of **thumb-in-palm deformity**, the thumb cannot be actively moved from palmar abduction to radial abduction, and passively only slightly (Fig. 5.10a, b). The base joint is in a flexed position, the palmar skin is significantly shortened. The end joint often stands in hyperextension in cases of long-term untreated thumb-in-palm deformity (Fig. 5.9a, b). There is an imbalance between the shortened flexors and the weak extensors. The muscles in the first interdigital fold and of the thenar (M. interosseus dorsalis I, M. adductor pollicis, M. flexor pollicis brevis, M. abductor pollicis brevis, M. opponens pollicis) can be significantly shortened and partly have fibrotic components (Chap. 1). The M. flexor pollicis longus is always shortened. If untreated, this malposition forces children to hold larger objects with both hands (Fig. 5.9c). In addition to manual treatment, a nightly splint therapy is recommended in infancy and toddlerhood. At this early age, the musculoskeletal system is still softer and more elastic than in older children, and the therapy is more successful. Early improvement of thumb mobility also promotes the child's development through the induction of neuronal connections (Chap. 1).

▶ A **fibrotic change** is a pathological change of the muscle tissue into connective tissue cells and collagen fibers.

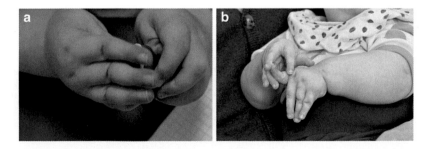

Fig. 5.8 a 22-month-old girl with Sheldon-Hall syndrome. When pressure is applied to an object, the proximal interphalangeal joints of the middle, index, and ring fingers of the right hand and the distal joint of the left thumb are hyperextended. **b** 10-month-old girl with Wieacker-Wolff syndrome. Fingers 2–4 are in windblown hand malposition, the thumbs show a thumb-in-palm deformity, and the proximal interphalangeal joints of D2–5 are hyperextendable. The index finger of the left hand is hyperextended by the infant with just slight pressure. (© Children's Hospital Wilhelmstift, with kind permission)

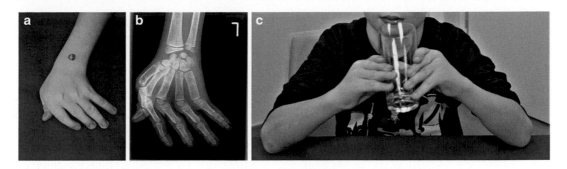

Fig. 5.9   a, b Photo and X-ray of an 8-year-old boy with Freeman-Sheldon syndrome. There is a severe thumb-in-palm deformity with hyperextension of the thumb's distal joint, a windblown hand deformity, and hyperextensibility of the proximal interphalangeal joints. **c** Due to the hand deformities, the boy can only grasp a narrow glass with both hands. (© Children's Hospital Wilhelmstift, with kind permission)

5.2   Motion Analysis

A motion analysis captures the affected regions, the extent of the deformities, and the existing strength of the patients. It is important to recognize the existing motor possibilities and the compensatory abilities of the children and to include them in the treatment.

5.2.1   Assessment of Altered Physiology in Infancy and Toddlerhood

An **assessment of altered physiology in infancy and toddlerhood** is carried out by observing the young patient and talking to the parents. They are asked about their child's

movements in everyday life in order to estimate the extent of the disease.

The older the child, the better activities and participation can be analyzed together with the child.

5.2.2   Analysis of Activities and Participation in Childhood

To obtain an accurate **analysis of activities and participation in childhood**, the PEAP (Pediatric Occupational Therapy Assessment and Process Instrument) (Kraus and Romein 2015) or the COSA (Child Occupational Self Assessment) (Kramer et al. 2021) can be used, among other things. These assessments not only give the therapist an overview of everyday

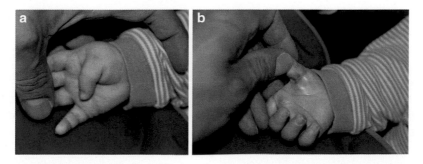

Fig. 5.10   a 10-week-old boy with a thumb-in-palm deformity. The thumb lies in the palm and cannot be actively extended from the palmar malposition. **b** When passively stretching the thumb, a significant shortening of the palmar soft tissues becomes visible. The shiny skin indicates significant tension in the area of the thumb base joint. The thumb can only be passively brought into extension to a limited extent. (© Children's Hospital Wilhelmstift, with kind permission)

problems, but also provide an overview of environmental factors and the patient's needs.

To avoid influencing the children, the parents and the child should be interviewed separately. At the very least, the parents should sit outside of their child's field of vision. For severely affected children, it quickly becomes clear that almost all areas in the PEAP or COSA are impaired in some form. Therefore, the assessment can help to initially focus on one area of activity or a specific task. In the PEAP, the fields of activity for children between 5–6 years and 7–8 years are pictured. It becomes clear: The more severe the arthrogryposis, the less the child can act independently. The various degrees of severity described on the previous pages can be rated in relation to everyday activities by patients and parents in the PEAP with

- no problem,
- minor problem,
- significant problem,
- major problem.

Secondly, the importance of the activity is rated:

- not important,
- somewhat important,
- important,
- very important.

The following areas are analyzed in the PEAP:

Self-sufficiency

- **Eating and Drinking**
  Taking food and drinks independently, bringing food to the mouth. This includes pouring something to drink, using cutlery, for example to spread butter on a bread or to cut something.
- **Dressing and Undressing**
  Putting on and taking off clothes independently, opening and closing buttons and zippers, independent dressing and undressing, also in sports.
- **Toilet Use**

Going to the toilet alone, dressing and undressing, cleaning the genital area, washing and drying hands.

- **Body Care**
  Washing face and hands, brushing teeth, applying toothpaste to toothbrush, combing hair. Beginning to shower or bathe independently, including washing hair.
- **Mobility**
  Moving to reach a goal, climbing stairs, riding a scooter or bicycle, using a wheelchair independently.

Productivity

- **Constructing**
  Playing with building blocks, plug-in blocks, working on a puzzle.
- **Tools**
  Using scissors to cut along a line, safe and measured pen guidance or using a glue stick.
- **Cultural Techniques**
  Writing letters, adequate pen holding, coloring or tracing
- **Completing Tasks**
  Helping at home or in the daycare, for example tidying up the room, setting the table, helping in the kitchen.
- **Interaction in the Group**
  Following rules, being considerate, reacting to instructions, actively participating in group activities.

Leisure and Play

- **Listening and Telling**
  Listening to and understanding stories, reporting experiences understandably.
- **Performing Physical Games**
  Actively participating in games, for example: climbing, throwing, catching, shooting, running, participating in sports.
- **Playing Together**
  Board or card games, video or computer games
- **Occupying Oneself Independently**

Moving around alone in the apartment to occupy oneself. Playing with cars, dolls, building blocks, painting.

- **Role-Playing**
  Slipping into an imagined role and filling it, with play materials and devices, such as playing house, building caves. Responding to the wishes of play partners.
  (Kraus and Romein 2015)

In severe forms of arthrogryposis, it is particularly important to recognize the needs of the children (Fig. 5.11). For this, the COSA (Child Occupational Self Assessment) can be used between the ages of 8 and 13.

In the COSA, activities are not summarized, but specifically asked about, such as: "I can wash myself alone".

The child can decide:

- I can't do this well at all.
- I can't do this very well.
- I can do this well.
- I can do this very well.

This is followed by how important it is for the child to be able to perform this activity:

- This is not important to me at all.
- This is not very important to me.
- This is important to me.
- This is very important to me.

From the discrepancy between what the child cannot do well at all and what is very important for the child, it is filtered which activities need to be specifically practiced or where there is still a need for medical aid provision.

Among other things, questions follow like:
"I can move as I want."
"I can use my hands well."
In total, the child evaluates 25 questions.
(Kramer et al. 2021).

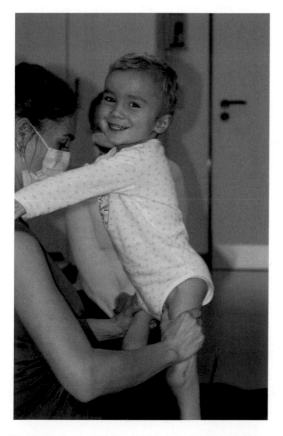

Fig. 5.11 3-year-old boy with a severe form of arthrogryposis multiplex congenita during motion analysis. The mother stabilizes her son's legs so that he can stand upright. The hypotrophic arms are positioned by the mother on her shoulders to provide him with support. This boy cannot stand up on his own due to weak musculature. (© Children's Hospital Wilhelmstift, with kind permission)

5.3 Treatments

After the analysis of body functions and structures, activities and participation, the corresponding treatment takes place.

All the therapy and treatment concepts described here refer to the upper extremities.

Interdisciplinary cooperation between doctors, therapists, orthopedic technicians, parents, and patients is important throughout the child's development. Treatment goals must be constantly reassessed and discussed during growth to achieve the greatest possible independence and satisfaction of the child.

The treatment goals are:

- Improvement of mobility,
- Improvement of joint position,
- Improvement of function and strength,
- the use of aids,
- satisfaction and independence of the child.

Daily training to maintain and ideally strengthen the muscles is especially necessary in severe forms of AMC. In addition, an aid and learning to use it promotes the child's development, independence, and thus satisfaction.

The goal of therapy is to improve functional limitations by improving position, strength, and mobility and to support helpful compensatory movements. This is intended to strengthen independence in everyday life.

▶ Even small improvements can be big steps for the patients.

5.3.1 Treatment Concept

1. From birth or from the time of diagnosis, treatment to strengthen the musculoskeletal system is very important. Parents must be intensively instructed in manual treatment and carry it out daily at home.
2. From the first weeks of life, thermoplastic splint therapy can support the manual treatment of the hands. The splints continuously stretch the joints, usually during night's sleep. The joint position is improved, thereby increasing the range of motion, mobility, and strength. The splint or orthotic therapy is continuously adapted to the age and severity of the disease.
3. To improve mobility, surgical interventions may be useful depending on the degree of contracture and functional restriction. Postoperatively, manual therapy must be resumed as soon as possible after consultation with the surgeon and temporarily intensified. In most cases, postoperative splint therapy is necessary to prevent recurrences and counteract scar traction.

4. Provision of aids is an important component. Through them the child becomes more independent and learns new gripping functions. The necessity and benefit should be regularly reviewed and adjusted in consultation with parents and child (at least every 2 years).
5. Freeman-Sheldon and Sheldon-Hall Syndrome are among the clinical disease patterns of syndromal arthrogryposis. There are similarities and differences between these syndromes in terms of joint malposition and soft tissue changes. Both manual therapy and splint treatment must therefore be individually adapted.

▶ Examples depending on the developmental and therapy status illustrate the treatment steps—see the end of the chapter.

5.3.2 Manual Therapy

In the manual treatment of children with arthrogryposis, the following factors should be considered: If only passive mobility is present, it must be maintained and improved. This allows the children to use their limbs as levers, for example to bring the hand to the mouth by pressing against the table edge. If active mobility is limited but possible, manual therapy is performed to improve both passive and active range of motion. Improving the passive range of motion is a prerequisite for improving active mobility. Due to the multiple joint malpositions, the therapist should analyze together with the parents which joints are most important for promoting independence and focus on these in the stretching treatment.

▶ To stretch tissue appropriately, the impulse on the structures must not be too weak. This stretch is held for about 10 to 20 seconds and repeated as often as possible. The stretching treatment should be carried out daily by the parents, and a splint treatment at night is advisable as a support.

5.3.2.1 Shoulder Joints

The **shoulder joints** do not need to be manually treated as often, as mobility is hardly restricted in most cases, and the extent of the movement restriction does not affect children in their daily lives. However, treatment of the shoulder may be necessary for children who are born with severe joint malpositions. Manual stretching of the shoulder and elbow is best performed in the supine position, but can also be done in a seated position for restless children. The parents' task is to distract the children.

Manual Stretching of the Shoulder

The directions of movement of the shoulder are:

- the anteversion and retroversion in the sagittal plane,
- the abduction and adduction in the frontal plane,
- the rotation in the horizontal plane.

The passive and active range of motion is checked before therapy. Restrictions of active shoulder mobility are visible as a protraction of the shoulder girdle, an internal rotation of the arms, and muscular atrophies. Treatment of the shoulder for passive movement improvement is only indicated if it does not decrease stability for the child. Children who cannot walk and move by sliding on their buttocks use their arms as support to lift their buttocks (Fig. 5.12a, b).

▶ A **protraction** is the forward movement of a body part e.g. shoulder blade or lower jaw.

The focus is on anteversion and abduction. These directions of movement are passively performed by the child in the lateral position or sitting by actively shifting the trunk.

- The therapist fixes the acromion from above with the holding hand,
- with the other hand, the humerus is grasped, the child's forearm rests on the therapist's forearm,
- the holding hand presses the shoulder girdle downwards,
- the active hand moves the arm into abduction or anteversion, depending on the movement restriction,
- the arm may need to be brought from internal rotation to the neutral position,
- if an elastic resistance is felt, the stretch is intensified and held at this position (Fig. 5.13a, b).

The improvement of the range of motion allows the child a larger radius of movement in space, which is automatically incorporated into everyday life.

> **Caution:**
> Treatment of the shoulder for passive movement improvement is only indicated if it does not decrease stability for the child.

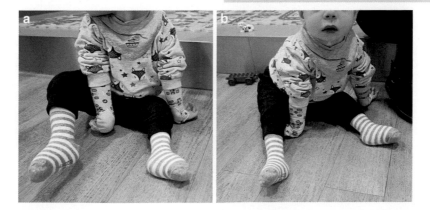

Fig. 5.12 **a** 1.5-year-old boy with a severe form of AMC. The boy pushes himself off the ground with the backs of his hands and can thus lift his buttocks to move forward. **b** The shoulder girdle is in clear protraction. (© Children's Hospital Wilhelmstift, with kind permission)

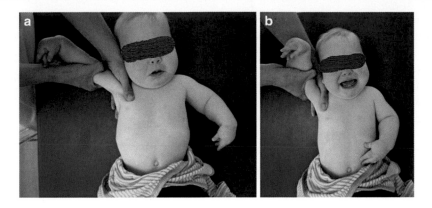

Fig. 5.13 **a** Stretching of the shoulder into abduction. **b** Stretching of the shoulder into anteversion. (© Children's Hospital Wilhelmstift, with kind permission)

5.3.2.2 Elbow

The passive flexion of the **elbows** is important for the child to be able to reach the mouth with the hand. If active mobility is restricted, children use the edge of the table or their knee as a lever to reach the mouth by bending the elbow joint.

Manual stretching of the elbow joint
The treatment includes:

- the therapist holds the upper arm near the joint with one hand and the forearm with the other hand (Fig. 5.14a),

- the elbow joint is passively guided into extension or flexion (Fig. 5.14b) depending on the restriction of movement,
- the proximal hand firmly grips the upper arm and holds it in a neutral position. The supine position facilitates therapy, as the upper arm can be fixed on a support.
- The distal hand is the action hand and guides the forearm into flexion and supination (Fig. 5.14b) or into extension and supination.

At the end of the movement, depending on the severity of the contracture, a hard or soft elastic

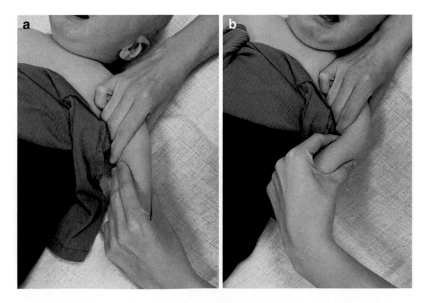

Fig. 5.14 **a** This boy has no active elbow mobility. The elbows are spontaneously in extension. To passively bend the joint, the lower and upper arm are grasped. **b** The arm is passively brought into flexion and held there. (© Children's Hospital Wilhelmstift, with kind permission)

stop is felt. At this point, the stretch should be slightly intensified and held. If resistance is felt, the stretch is intensified, held for at least 10 to 20 seconds, and the movement is repeated as often as possible, but at least 10 times. The stretching exercises must be performed daily at home by the parents.

5.3.2.3 Wrists

The **wrists** in arthrogryposis are often in strong palmar flexion and also little stretchable passively. Due to the contracted joint position, even infants have difficulty supporting themselves on their hands in the prone position or crawling. Also, for many gripping functions, the optimal powerful wrist position is a dorsal extension of about 40° (Chap. 1). Therefore, the manual treatment of the wrists is of very high importance in the treatment of AMC children.

Manual stretching of the wrist

In case of flexion contracture, the following procedure is used:

- With one hand, the distal forearm is palpated and with the other hand, the palm of the hand (Fig. 5.15a).
- The hand on the child's forearm is the holding hand, the hand on the palm at the level of the base joints is the action hand.
- Once the structures are firmly gripped, the wrist is moved out of an existing ulnar deviation (Fig. 5.15a).
- With the action hand, the wrist is gently stretched dorsally by slight traction (Fig. 5.15b, c).

It is important that the therapist firmly grips the palm of the hand, not the fingers, otherwise the base joints will be stretched too much into hyperextension. If resistance is felt, the stretch is held and the exercise is repeated several times.

Extension contracture

In children with Freeman-Sheldon and Sheldon-Hall syndrome, in addition to the deformities of the fingers, there may be extension contractures of the wrists. These significantly restrict the dynamic use of the hand in everyday life. The gripping technique is the same as for the flexion contracture. The child's hand is moved out of ulnar deviation and gently stretched palmarly by slight traction and held there. If resistance is felt, the stretch is held and the exercise is repeated several times. If necessary, additional treatment can be done with a flexion splint.

5.3.2.4 Fingers 2–5

In children with arthrogryposis, the **fingers 2–5** are usually in a neutral position at the base joints, sometimes in ulnar deviation, occasionally also in hyperextension, less often in flexion. Active movement is often only abduction and adduction at the base joints. Passively, the base joints can only be stretched into flexion to a limited extent. The middle and end joints often show flexion contractures. The intrinsic musculature is atrophied, therefore flattened. The mobility of the finger joints varies from child to child. Overall, active mobility is usually severely limited. Therefore, children often use the pinch grip or side grip (Chap. 1).

Many children also have a thumb-in-palm deformity. The different malpositions of the

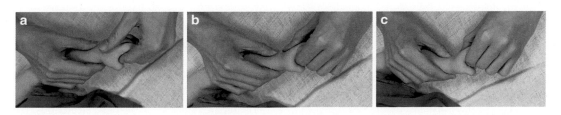

Fig. 5.15 a–c The wrist is first moved out of ulnar deviation, then the wrist is gently stretched into the best possible extension. (© Children's Hospital Wilhelmstift, with kind permission)

fingers require different manual techniques. A detailed functional analysis must be carried out before starting exercises. The focus of manual treatment is on the joints that have a contracture.

Manual stretching of fingers 2–5
Treatment of the base joints to improve flexion:
The base joints are grasped close to the joint. In this case:

- the proximal hand of the therapist is the holding hand. It fixes the metacarpal bone of the affected finger at the level of the head proximal to the base joint in a sandwich grip.
- The distal hand of the therapist is the action hand. The therapist's index finger is placed dorsally at the level of the head of the base phalanx.
- The action hand applies pressure dorsally to the base phalanx head and brings the base joint into maximum flexion.

If there is an elastic resistance, the stretch is intensified and then held.

Stretching of the middle joints into extension

- the proximal hand of the therapist is the holding hand. It fixes the base joint in a sandwich grip from the palmar and dorsal side.
- The distal hand of the therapist is the action hand. It fixes the affected finger of the child dorsally with the index finger at the level of the base phalanx head and palmarly with the thumb at the level of the middle phalanx.
- The action hand maximally stretches the middle joint by applying pressure dorsally to the base phalanx head and palmarly to the middle phalanx.

If an elastic resistance is felt, the stretch is intensified and then held.
Since both the middle and the end joints often not only have an extension deficit but also a flexion deficit, the manual treatment must also take place in flexion.

Stretching of the middle joints into flexion
The middle joints are grasped close to the joint, in this case:

- the proximal hand of the therapist is the holding hand. It fixes the base joint of the affected finger proximal to the middle joint in a sandwich grip.
- The distal hand of the therapist is the action hand. The therapist's index finger is placed dorsally proximal to the end joint on the middle phalanx head.
- The action hand applies pressure dorsally to the middle phalanx head and brings the middle joint into maximum flexion.

If an elastic resistance is felt, the stretch is intensified and then held.
Stretching of the end joints into extension:
In case of flexion contractures in the end joint, the procedure is the same as for stretching the middle joints, only:

- the holding hand fixes the middle and the base joint,
- the index finger of the action hand is placed dorsally on the middle phalanx head and palmarly on the child's fingertip.
- By applying pressure dorsally to the middle phalanx head and pressure palmarly to the fingertip, the end joint is stretched into the best possible extension.

Stretching of the end joints into flexion
The therapist's holding hand fixes the palm from the ulnar side and holds the affected finger in extension at the base joint. The action hand presses the end phalanx of the finger towards the base phalanx into the small fist.

5.3.2.5 Thumb
The manual treatment of the **thumb** in a thumb-in-palm deformity is a special case. It is important during the entire stretching process that the base joint of the thumb is not stretched into hyperextension. Constant stretching into

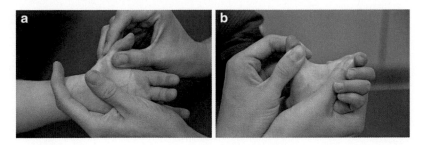

Fig. 5.16 **a** The thumb is led out of the palmar abduction. The thumb's base joint is supported from the dorsal side to prevent hyperextension. **b** Through a flowing movement from the index finger base joint to the thumb tip, the thumb is led into the maximum radial abduction. Here too, the thumb's base joint is supported from the dorsal side. (© Children's Hospital Wilhelmstift, with kind permission)

hyperextension would lead to instability in the base joint.

Stretching of the thumb into radial and palmar abduction:

- the therapist's holding hand fixes the palm in the area of the hand edge,
- the therapist's action hand grips with the thumb at the level of the saddle joint/thenar muscles of the child. Now the therapist strokes with pressure from the saddle joint over the base phalanx to proximal of the end joint (Fig. 5.16a). In this way, the thumb is stretched into the best possible palmar and radial abduction. The stretch is held for 20 s and repeated several times, e.g., after each diaper change.
- With the index and middle fingers of the action hand, the thumb is fixed from the dorsal side, thus preventing hyperextension in the base joint. The index finger is located distal to the base joint, the middle finger proximal (Fig. 5.16a).
- At the same time, the thumb of the action hand should stretch the child's saddle joint into the best possible radial abduction by the therapist not only stroking over the thenar muscles towards the end joint, but also stretching away from the second metacarpal bone into radial abduction (Fig. 5.16b).

Caution:
The base joint of the thumb must not be stretched into hyperextension. This would lead to palmar instability in this joint.

5.3.3 Splint and Orthosis Therapy

The **splint and orthosis therapy** starts from the first months of life. In most cases, finger and wrist joints are treated with splints. An elbow splint is indicated in the case of a rapidly deteriorating contracture of the elbow joint. Through splinting and manual therapy, surgery can usually be avoided, or at least the procedure can be simplified. Both therapies are helpful in preparation for surgery. Postoperatively, splints and orthoses can maintain and possibly even improve the surgical result. They are individually adjusted, and their benefit is regularly reviewed in consensus with the treating physicians, parents, and patients. The following describes different types of splints and orthoses based on various findings.

Caution:
Splints and orthoses, especially in infancy and early childhood, must exert very little pressure on the tissue. The pressure must be well distributed to prevent soft tissue compression. Children with arthrogryposis have few solid structures due to the underdeveloped, remodeled muscles.

5.3.3.1 Elbow

Static Elbow Splint
This type of orthosis is used for the treatment of both flexion and extension contractures (Fig. 5.17a, b). The prerequisite is that the elbow

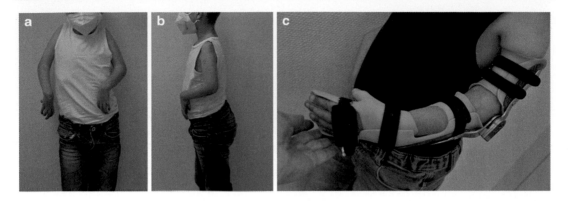

Fig. 5.17 a, b 7-year-old boy with pronounced hypoplasia of the entire musculature of the upper extremities. There is a flexion contracture of the elbow joints, 60° on the left and 75° on the right. Passive flexion is possible up to 140°. The hand and finger joints are in a flexion contracture. **c** With the static elbow-Quengel orthosis, the elbow joint is extended. At the same time, it holds the wrist and finger joints in the best possible extension and the thumb in the best possible palmar and radial abduction. This splint is worn at night with moderate stretching and during the day for short intervals with maximum stretching. (© Children's Hospital Wilhelmstift, with kind permission)

joints can be passively stretched. To achieve the greatest possible effect, this orthosis should be worn overnight with a moderate stretch. The splint therapy is supplemented by short exercise intervals during the day with a strong stretch up to the pain threshold.

This orthosis

- improves elbow mobility in flexion and extension.
  Depending on the need
- the wrist is kept in the best possible extension,
- the palm is stretched,
- fingers 2 to 5 are kept in the best possible extension and splinted away from a possibly existing deviation position,
- the thumb is splinted in the best possible palmar and radial adduction,
- it is used postoperatively after arthrolysis and tendon lengthening.

The plaster cast is made, if possible, in a neutral position of the distal and proximal radioulnar joint and in 90° or the best possible flexion of the elbow. The wrist is cast in the best possible extension. The orthosis can also include the fingers if necessary. The orthosis splints the arm on the palmar side and ends, depending on what is needed, distal to the wrist, the palm, or at the fingertips. The orthosis covers about 2/3 of the length of the upper arm, without restricting shoulder mobility. The straps are applied over a large area so that the pressure is distributed and the arm is adequately fixed in the orthosis during the splinting. The area of the crook of the arm is left out in the orthosis to allow movements (Fig. 5.17c). It is recommended to raise the material there (Chap. 8) to avoid pinching and to guide the soft tissue. If the elbow joints are stiff, this orthosis is used postoperatively after capsulotomy.

Caution:
The static elbow Quengel splint can be used from about the third year of life. It is absolutely necessary to ensure that the child does not perform any evasive movements in the shoulder while using the splint. The weight of the splint and the pull into flexion can lead to an increase in the protraction of the shoulder girdle. If this is the case, the splint should initially be avoided and manual stretching should be the primary treatment.

Postoperative use after arthrolysis of the elbow joint and tendon lengthening

After surgery, the static elbow Quengel splint supports manual treatment. It gradually stretches the operated muscles and tendons through long stretching. The elbow joint is alternately held in the best possible flexion and extension in the orthosis. Intensive manual treatment and orthosis therapy prevent adhesions and re-stiffening.

Static Elbow Quengel Orthosis

- **Arm position in the orthosis:**

  The upper arm is enclosed up to 2/3 of its length, without restricting shoulder mobility.

  The forearm is in the neutral-zero position.

  The wrist is in the best possible pain-free extension.

  If necessary, fingers 2–5 are enclosed in the best possible extension. If there is a compensatory hyperextension in the base joints 2–5, these are splinted in 10–20° flexion. The thumb is in the best possible palmar and radial abduction.

- **Orthosis enclosure:**

  From the palm to the upper arm in a half-shell with circular cutout around the elbow.

  The hand, forearm, and upper arm are enclosed circularly or with wide straps to ensure hold during the stretching.

  At the proximal upper arm, the orthosis is as long as possible without restricting shoulder movements.

  Fingers 2–5 are individually enclosed from the palmar side. This can compensate for different contractures. A pressure pad at the level of the dorsal base phalanges fixes the fingers in the orthosis.

  The thumb receives a palmar and ulnar guide or is enclosed circularly.

  Windows for skin ventilation, depending on the size of the child and soft tissue condition.

- **Pressure points:**

  Palmar side: upper arm, forearm, and palm—armpit and elbow are spared

  Dorsal side: firm straps over the entire length of the splint

  Radial side: guide in the half-shells for the upper arm, forearm to second metacarpal bone or index finger tip

  Ulnar side: guide in the half-shells upper arm, forearm to fifth metacarpal bone or little finger tip

  The thumb receives a guide from the palmar and ulnar side

- **Recommended materials** (Chap. 8):
  - Streifi-Flex
  - Carbon brace
  - Deflector
  - Strap with Velcro fastener
  - Finger pad
  - Static dynamic joint

▶ **Caution:**

The edges in the area of the elbow and at the proximal end of the splint must be generously raised because of the soft tissue displacement (Chap. 8). Only at the level of the armpit does the splint material rest on the upper arm to avoid chafing on the thorax.

This splint is used for the treatment of contractures and after surgeries. Conservative therapy prevents a worsening of the contracture and improves it in many cases. Postoperatively, it supports manual treatment by alternately stretching the operated structures in flexion and extension.

5.3.3.2 Wrist

Forearm Splint with Palm and Thumb Enclosure

A thermoplastic night splint can be made to stretch the wrist, palm, and thumb (Fig. 5.18b). This splint is suitable when the fingers have only very minor contractures and the focus is on the flexion contracture of the wrist (Fig. 5.18a). Since in many cases a thumb-in-palm deformity

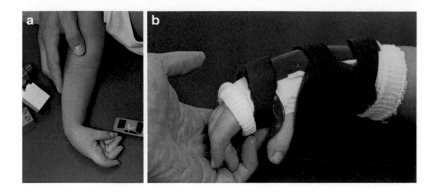

Fig. 5.18 **a** The wrist is spontaneously in 60° flexion. **b** The thermoplastic night splint stretches the wrist, thumb, and palm. (© Kinderkrankenhaus Wilhelmstift, with kind permission)

is present and the palm also shows a shortening, these are included in the splint.

The forearm orthosis

- keeps the wrist in the best possible extension and counteracts an existing deviation,
- stretches the palm,
- keeps the thumb in the best possible palmar and radial abduction

This splint serves as a night splint.

To prevent the arm from being levered out of the splint in the case of a pronounced flexion contracture, a dorsal cover is useful (Fig. 5.18b). The splint is modeled from the palmar side around the ulnar edge of the hand to the dorsal side and encompasses the entire forearm, the palm, and the back of the hand. The pressure is thus distributed over a large area. To avoid pressure points on the dorsal side of the wrist and the ulnar head, a pad is glued to prominent areas before modeling. After removal of the pad, a small space remains for the carpus and the ulnar head.

▶ This splint can be used from about the third year of life.

This type of thermoplastic splint can be **slightly modified** to be useful from the first weeks of life to support manual therapy. Thus, intensive stretching of the wrist, palm, and thumb can begin in infancy (Fig. 5.19b). If the fingers are

also severely affected, they can be integrated into the splint (Fig. 5.19a). However, since modeling the splint material in such small children, especially with varying degrees of finger contractures, is difficult, the focus can first be placed on the wrist, the palm, and the thumb (Fig. 5.19c). The dorsal cover is replaced by padded straps to facilitate the insertion of the small hand.

▶ This splint can be used from the first weeks of life.

Postoperative Use after Carpal Wedge Osteotomy
Forearm splint with palmar inclusion during the K-wire fixation:

If a splint is made after a surgical straightening of the wrist, the carpal wedge osteotomy, Velcro fasteners fix the arm in the splint (Fig. 5.21a, b). In this case, the hand can be placed more easily into the splint, which is particularly useful shortly after the operation to avoid pain. The inserted K-wires fix the wrist (Fig. 5.20). In this case, the splint must definitely include the metacarpophalangeal joints to give the surgical area the necessary rest for healing and to protect the joint-fixing K-wires. If the metacarpophalangeal joints continue to hyperextend (Fig. 5.21a, b), they are gently exercised manually every day. The fingers are not yet included shortly after the operation, as the child wears the splint permanently and the use of the fingers should remain possible.

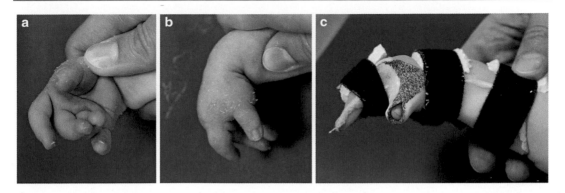

Fig. 5.19 **a**, **b** 4-week-old girl. The wrist is spontaneously in 90° flexion and can be passively stretched to 40° flexion. The fingers show different flexion contractures and the thumb a thumb-in-palm deformity. The palm is shortened. **c** The thermoplastic night splint stretches the wrist, the palm, the thumb, and the fingers. On the dorsal side, the soft tissue is slightly compressed by the extension of the wrist. Padded Velcro straps fix the hand and forearm in the splint. The padding prevents pressure points on the delicate compressed skin that can be caused by the Velcro strap. (© Kinderkrankenhaus Wilhelmstift, with kind permission)

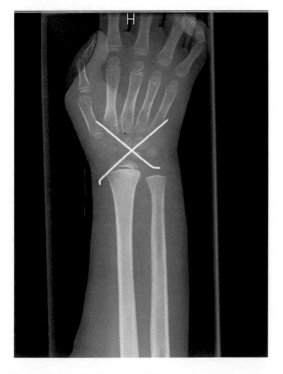

Fig. 5.20 K-wire fixation of the carpus and wrist after carpal wedge osteotomy in a 5-year-old patient. (© Children's Hospital Wilhelmstift, with kind permission)

Postoperative Use after Carpal Wedge Osteotomy
Forearm splint with palm inclusion after removal of the K-wires:

After the removal of the K-wires, the wrist is placed in the best possible extension in the splint. If the child still has to wear the splint continuously, it receives a forearm splint with palm inclusion (Fig. 5.21a, b). If the splint is uscd as a night splint, the child receives a splint with palm inclusion, additionally with thumb inclusion or an orthosis with individual finger inclusion (Fig. 5.22b).

Forearm splint with palm and thumb inclusion
- **Hand position of the holder:**
  Hand 1: Fingers 2–5 are pulled distally. The therapist's thumb is used as counterpressure on the wrist or the back of the hand
  Hand 2: fixes the upper arm with thumb pressure at the elbow, the elbow joint is

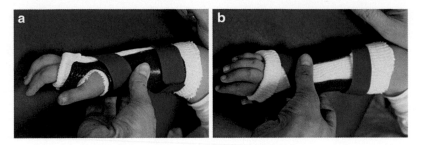

Fig. 5.21   a, b The same boy with a thermoplastic forearm splint with palm inclusion for fixation of the wrist after carpal wedge osteotomy and K-wire fixation. The fingers are not included during the time of K-wire fixation to allow their movement. The metacarpophalangeal joints of fingers 2–5 are included from the palmar side in the splint to ensure sufficient immobilization. (© Children's Hospital Wilhelmstift, with kind permission)

extended, this position serves as counterpressure for Hand 1
- **Pressure points of the splint:**
  Radial side = from the proximal forearm to the metacarpophalangeal joint of the index finger
  Ulnarside = from the proximal forearm to the metacarpophalangeal joint of the little finger
  Palmar side = from the metacarpophalangeal joints 2–5 to the proximal forearm
  Dorsal side = proximal forearm to proximal of the metacarpophalangeal joints
  Thumb = from the palmar and ulnar side

Forearm Splint with Thumb and Finger Enclosure
- **Hand position of the holder:**
  Hand 1: Fingers 2–5 are pulled distally by the therapist's fingers. The therapist's thumb provides counterpressure on the wrist
  Hand 2: fixes the upper arm with thumb pressure on the elbow, the elbow is extended, this position serves as counterpressure for Hand 1
- **Pressure points of the splint:**
  Radial side = from the proximal forearm to the tip of the index finger
  Ulnar side = from the proximal forearm to the tip of the little finger

Palmar side = from the fingertips 2–5 to the proximal forearm
Dorsal side = proximal forearm to proximal of the metacarpophalangeal joints
Thumb = from the palmar and ulnar side

Postoperative Splint after Carpal Wedge Osteotomy
Forearm splint with palm enclosure during K-wire fixation

- **Hand position of the holder:**
  Hand 1: fixes fingers 2–5, they are gently pulled distally
  Hand 2: fixes the upper arm with thumb pressure on the elbow, the elbow is extended and gently held, the K-wire determines the wrist position, therefore stretching of the wrist is not possible
- **Pressure points of the splint:**
  Radial side = from the proximal forearm to distal of the metacarpophalangeal joint of the index finger
  Ulnar side = from the proximal forearm to distal of the metacarpophalangeal joint of the little finger
  Palmar side = distal of the metacarpophalangeal joints 2–5 to the proximal forearm
  Dorsal side = Fleece straps fix the hand and forearm in the splint

Thumb = remains free

If this splint is used **postoperatively after carpal wedge osteotomy and removal of the K-wires**, the wrist is straightened into the best possible extension.

- **Recommended materials** (Chap. 8):
  - Thermoplastic material 2.0 mm or 3.2 mm
  - Tubular bandage 2.5 or 5 cm wide
  - Velcro strap
  - Fleece strap
  - Edge padding
  - Possibly padding between the splint edges

Caution:

Avoid deviation and hyperextension in the metacarpophalangeal joints. Encase lax finger joints in approx. 20° flexion. Due to soft tissue displacement, joints often appear hyperextended. For safety, the position of the joints should be checked by palpation.

5.3.3.3 Wrist, Fingers and Thumb

Forearm Orthosis with Individual Finger Enclosure

This orthosis is made by orthopedic technicians after a plaster cast. The wrist is splinted in the best possible extension, the middle and end joints in 0° and the base joints in slight flexion or 0°. The thumb is stretched in the best possible palmar and radial abduction. This orthosis is used postoperatively and in conservative treatment (Fig. 5.22a) from the sixth month of life as a night orthosis. Both the wrist, all fingers and the palm are stretched in this orthosis (Fig. 5.22b).

The forearm orthosis

- keeps the wrist in the best possible extension and removes any existing ulnar abduction.
  If there is an extension contracture of the wrist, it is splinted up to a maximum of 0°.
- stretches the palm,
- keeps the thumb in radial abduction, the end joint is in slight flexion of approx. 20°, especially in case of existing hypermobility,

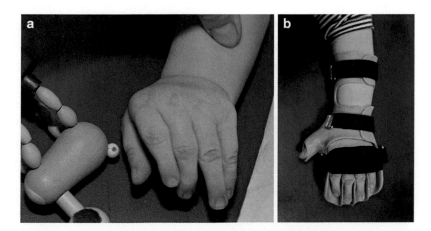

Fig. 5.22 **a** One-year-old boy with lax ligaments, a windblown hand and a thumb-in-palm deformity. The wrist is in extension contracture. **b** Streifi-Flex orthosis with individual finger inclusion, fixation of the wrist in 20° extension, out of the pre-existing extension contracture of 40°. The metacarpophalangeal and middle joints are splinted in 20° flexion, the index finger is still in a slight ulnar deviation in the splint, fingers 3–5 could be completely straightened out of their ulnar deviation, the thumb is in the best possible palmar and radial abduction. (© Children's Hospital Wilhelmstift, with kind permission)

- encloses fingers 2 to 5 in the best possible extension and corrects an ulnar abduction. If the base joints are hyperextended, they are encased in approx. 20° flexion. If the middle joints have lax ligaments, they are also splinted in approx. 20° flexion.

These orthoses are applied before going to sleep.

▶ This splint can be used from about the sixth month of life.

Postoperative Care after palmar release of the long fingers through skin extension in the palm

If a palmar release with skin extension in the area of the palm and full-thickness skin grafting was performed to improve finger extension (Fig. 5.23a, b), a forearm orthosis with individual finger encasement is fitted after wound healing. Before fitting, the scars and especially the full-thickness skin graft should be examined to integrate a compression treatment (Chap. 6) into the orthosis therapy, if necessary. With additional compression treatment, the distance between the orthosis and the hand must be greater. This distance can be created during the making of the plaster cast for the plaster model with double-layered tubular bandages (Fig. 5.24).

Often, an operative palmar release can be prevented by early manual treatment and splint therapy in infancy or toddler age.

Forearm orthosis with individual finger encasement

- **Hand and finger position in the orthosis:**
  Wrist – best possible straightening to an extension up to 30°, in case of an extension contracture the wrist is straightened up to a maximum of 0°.
  Fingers 2–5 – Stretching of all base, middle and end joints (up to a maximum of 0° / with lax joints in approx. 20° flexion).
  Thumb – Stretching in palmar and radial abduction.
- **Orthosis encasement:**
  At least 1/2 of the circumference of forearm and hand are encased, orthosis length at least 2/3 of the forearm up to approx. 1 cm above the fingertips (due to growth). The thumb is encased approx. by 2/3 or completely enclosed.
- **Pressure points:**
  Palmar side: forearm to fingertips. Finger flexion contractures are compensated from the palmar side by the orthosis, the thumb is stretched out of the malposition by pressure from the palmar and ulnar side.
- Dorsal: firm pad at the level of the wrist, holder on the proximal forearm,

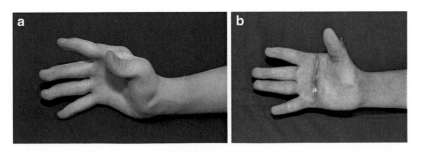

Fig. 5.23 a 8-year-old boy with shortened flexors of thumb and fingers, significant skin tension in the palm and in the area of the thumb base joint. All fingers can neither be fully extended actively nor passively. The thumb base joint is in flexion, the thumb end joint in compensatory hyperextension. **b** 6 weeks postoperatively after palmar release of fingers 2–5 through skin extension in the palm with full-thickness skin grafts. Straightening of the thumb by temporary K-wire fixation. (© Children's Hospital Wilhelmstift, with kind permission)

finger pad between base and middle joints.
- **Recommended materials** (Chap. 8):
  - Streifi-Flex
  - Carbon brace (if necessary)
  - Deflector
  - Strap with Velcro fastener
  - Finger pad

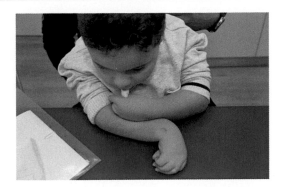

Fig. 5.24 5-year-old boy with a severe form of AMC. The entire musculature is hypotrophic, the shoulders show adduction and internal rotation, the elbows can be flexed passively, but not actively. The forearms are in pronation, the wrists in flexion, the thumbs show a thumb-in-palm deformity, the fingers are flexed, the palm is shortened. (© Children's Hospital Wilhelmstift, with kind permission)

Cave:

Avoid deviation and hyperextension in the finger base joints, with lax finger joints on the palmar side these should be encased in 10–20° flexion.

Static wrist Quengel-orthosis with individual finger encasement

This wrist quengel orthosis stretches the fingers, the palm, and the wrist at night (Fig. 5.24). In addition, it is used during the day as an exercise orthosis for maximum stretching of the wrist. During the night, the joint is extended or flexed until a stretch, but no pain, is felt. During the day, short exercise sessions are carried out, stretching the wrist for a few minutes to half an hour until the pain threshold is reached (Fig. 5.25a–c). These exercise sessions should be repeated several times a day.

This orthosis:

- improves active and passive wrist extension,
- stretches the palm,
- corrects an existing deviation of fingers 2 to 5 and keeps them in the best possible extension,
- keeps the thumb in the best possible palmar and radial abduction,
- serves as preparation for a carpal wedge osteotomy.

Due to a strong contracture of the wrist, the hand and forearm easily move out of the orthosis during treatment. This is prevented by a firm and wide fixation distal and proximal to

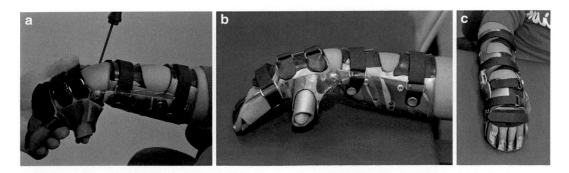

Fig. 5.25 **a–c** Static wrist quengel orthosis made of Streifi-Flex and carbon. The quengel joint brings the wrist into extension, the individual finger enclosure with the dorsal pad presses the fingers into the splint, the thumb is splinted from the palmar and ulnar side. The wrist is pressed into maximum extension several times a day for a maximum of 30 minutes. (© Children's Hospital Wilhelmstift, with kind permission)

the wrist. The fingers receive individual finger enclosures from the palmar side and a pad from the dorsal side. This fixes the fingers in the splint at the level of the base phalanx. The thumb is enclosed on the palmar and ulnar side. The stretching is done slowly and depends on the child's reaction (Fig. 5.25a–c).

By pressing into extension, the soft tissues on the dorsal wrist are compressed (Fig. 5.26b). Therefore, the orthosis material must be raised dorsally to guide the soft tissues (Chap. 8). Generous removal of the material is not recommended due to the changed soft tissue structure. In infancy (Fig. 5.26a), excessive compression of the soft tissues can be prevented by a cuff made of elastic, gently compressing fabric (Fig. 5.26c–e) (Chap. 8). To guide the thumb when inserting it into the splint, the thumb cuff can be left long there (Fig. 5.26c–e). The fingers are placed in the splint without pressure in wrist flexion. During the stretching of the wrist, the fingers are automatically stretched more and are slightly pushed distally.

This type of orthosis can also be used with minor modifications for wrist flexion in the case of an extension contracture. In this case, the splint material must be generously cut out on the palmar side proximal and distal to the wrist to allow flexion. Here too, the wide straps over the back of the hand and fingers and a fully enclosed thumb have proven effective in preventing the hand from evading the orthosis.

In most cases, an additional distal finger pad is needed dorsally of the middle joints to ensure the fingers are fully secured in the splint and do not escape.

▶ This splint can be used from about the sixth month of life.

Static Wrist-Quengel Orthosis with Individual Finger Enclosure
- **Hand position in the orthosis:**
  The hand and fingers rest in relaxed flexion in the orthosis, the wrist is taken out of its lateral deviation. The thumb is in the best possible abduction and retroversion.
- **Orthosis enclosure:**
  Palmar, radial and ulnar side in a half shell, with free space circularly around the wrist.
  The forearm is encased circularly or dorsally with wide straps to ensure fixation during treatment in the orthosis.
  The hand and thumb are enclosed circularly to prevent evasive movements.
  The fingers receive individual finger enclosure from the palmar side, which can treat different contractures of the finger joints. A pressure pad from the dorsal side fixes the fingers at the level of the base joints.

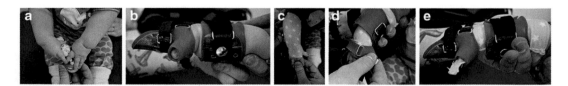

Fig. 5.26 **a** 7-month-old girl (same girl as in Fig. 5.19a–c). After 6 months of treatment, the wrists are spontaneously in 50° flexion, they can be actively stretched to 30° flexion and passively to 10° flexion. The thumbs can be moved more actively into palmar and radial abduction and the fingers can be fully extended. The fist closure is still restricted. Dorsally at the wrist, the soft tissues bulge due to the flexion contractures. **b** Static wrist quengel orthosis made of Streifi-Flex and carbon. The prominent soft tissues are compressed during the wrist straightening. They run the risk of being squeezed. **c** A custom-made compressive cuff is pulled over the palm, thumb, and entire forearm. **d** By leaving a long cuff on the thumb, it can easily be inserted into the splint. **e** The cuff compresses the tissue evenly. This reduces the compression of the dorsal soft tissues during treatment. (© Children's Hospital Wilhelmstift, with kind permission)

- **Pressure points:**
  Palmar side: forearm and entire hand, including the thumb
  Dorsal side: solid strap over the entire forearm length or two solid straps on the distal and proximal forearm and on the back of the hand, a dorsal pad over the finger base joints
  Ulnar side: thumb over its entire ulnar length
- **Recommended materials** (Chap. 8):
  - Streifi-Flex
  - Carbon brace
  - Deflector
  - Strap with Velcro fastener
  - Finger pad
  - Static dynamic joint, in very small children joints are used for the treatment of fingers

Caution:

If the wrist is extended in the orthosis, there is automatically a stronger stretching of the fingers in the orthosis. Therefore, they must be encased in a relaxed position in wrist flexion.

The edges in the area of the dorsal wrist must be generously raised due to the soft tissue displacement

▶ In infancy and toddler age, a joint for the treatment of fingers is used as a static-dynamic joint for the wrist. The usual dynamic joints are too large for the small arms (Chap. 8).

5.3.3.4 Thumb

Forearm Splint with Thumb Enclosure
If there is a sole thumb-in-palm deformity (Fig. 5.27a), a thermoplastic night splint is useful in infancy alongside manual therapy. The thumb is stretched in the splint in the best possible radial and palmar abduction. The base and end joint of the thumb must not be overstretched. The splint extends to the tip of the thumb to fully stretch the thumb and avoid pressure points at the tip of the thumb. The base joints of the other fingers are also included to stretch the entire thenar musculature. Enclosing one third to half of the forearm is necessary to guide the saddle joint into radial abduction and to better fix the splint, especially in infancy and early childhood. (Fig. 5.27b, c).

The forearm orthosis

- stretches the palm,
- keeps the thumb in the best possible palmar and radial abduction

This splint serves as a night splint in purely conservative treatment or postoperatively after a

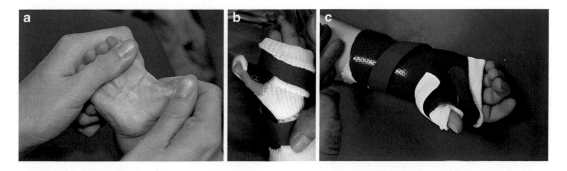

Fig. 5.27 **a** 7-month-old boy with a thumb-in-palm deformity. During passive stretching, a clear soft tissue tension of the entire palm and especially over the thumb base joint is noticeable. **b** 4-month-old boy. The thermoplastic night splint stretches the thumb into the best possible palmar and radial abduction and maximally opens the palm. **c** 6-year-old boy. The thermoplastic forearm splint counteracts a recurrence. (© Children's Hospital Wilhelmstift, with kind permission)

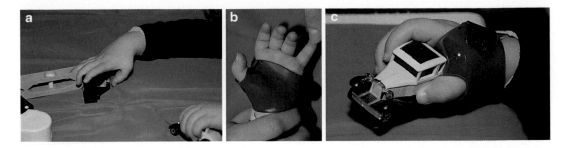

Fig. 5.28 **a** 20-month-old boy with a thumb-in-palm deformity. The thumb can be actively extended out of the palm. The child positions the base joints of fingers 2–5 in hyperextension and the wrist in flexion to compensate for the malposition. **b** A palm orthosis with thumb enclosure stabilizes the thumb base joint in a functional position, all joints except the thumb base and saddle joints remain free. **c** The stabilization of the thumb base joint improves the gripping function. The compensatory hyperextension of the base finger joints and the flexion of the wrist are no longer necessary. (© Children's Hospital Wilhelmstift, with kind permission)

release of the thumb as a day and night splint. At the same time, hypertrophic scars can be treated with a compression glove. The splint also supports manual treatment in the case of an emerging recurrence. Depending on the findings and the child's age, a thermoplastic C-splint or a forearm splint with or without inclusion of the finger base joints is sufficient.

In severe cases, a **thumb palm orthosis** made of Streifi-Flex or silicone can be made from the crawling age onwards (Fig. 5.28b, c). During the day, this orthosis straightens the thumb to facilitate gripping (Fig. 5.28a, c). Due to the corrected thumb position, the thumb is automatically stretched by the child's own weight when crawling.

The material must be stable enough to straighten the thumb and at the same time elastic enough to allow gripping. With the exception of the thumb base and saddle joints, all other joints in the orthosis are freely movable.

Forearm Splint with Thumb Enclosure
- **Hand position of the holder:**
  Hand 1: Fingers 2–5 are pulled distally and dorsally. The therapist's thumb holds the back of the hand to better extend the wrist
  Hand 2: fixes the proximal forearm and the elbow on the table

- **Pressure points of the splint:**
  Radial side = from the proximal forearm to the base joint of the index finger
  Ulnar side = from the proximal forearm to the base joint of the little finger
  Palmar side = from the base joints of fingers 2–5 to the proximal forearm
  Dorsal side = proximal forearm to proximal of the base joints of the fingers
  Thumb = from the palmar and ulnar side
- **Recommended materials** (Chap. 8):
  – Thermoplastic material 2.0 mm or 3.2 mm
  – Tubular bandage 2.5 or 5 cm wide
  – Velcro strap
  – Fleece strap
  – Edge padding
  – Possibly padding between the splint edges

This splint is also used postoperatively after a surgical release of the thumb.

Thumb Palm Orthosis
- **Hand and finger position in the splint:**
  Thumb – Stabilization of the first metacarpal and the thumb base joint in abduction and retroversion, but only so

far that opposition to the other fingers is still possible.

Palm – the palm is enclosed and slightly stretched

- **Splint enclosure:**
  The hand is fully encompassed, without restricting the movement of the base joints 2 to 5 and the wrist.
  The thumb base joint is fully encompassed, the end joint retains free mobility.
- **Pressure points:**
  Palmar side: edge of the hand and metacarpal bones up to distal of the thumb base joint
  Dorsal side: back of the hand
- **Recommended materials** (Chap. 8):
  - Streifi-Flex or
  - Silicone

> **Caution:**
> Deteriorations are possible during growth and likely during a growth spurt. They can usually be treated with conservative therapy. Therefore, regular growth checks are sensible.

5.3.4 Surgical Therapy

Children and parents must know that postoperative intensive manual treatment and splint therapy are necessary to maintain the achieved surgical result, to stretch soft tissues and scar tissue, and possibly to learn new movement sequences. The goal is to prevent a renewed stiffening of the joints and a weakening of the existing musculature. Therefore, postoperative care must be closely coordinated with the treating physician.

5.3.4.1 Elbow

Elbow Extension Contracture
If hand-mouth contact is not possible due to an elbow extension contracture, passive elbow mobility can be established by lengthening the triceps tendon and dorsal capsulotomy (Waters and Bae 2012).

Elbow Flexion Contracture
Here, the indication for surgery lies in the bothering extension deficit of the elbow. By lengthening the shortened elbow flexors and a ventral capsulotomy of the elbow joint, an improvement or establishment of passive elbow extension is achieved.

> **Caution:**
> If the operation makes hand-mouth contact difficult for the child, this operation is questioned.

5.3.4.2 Wrist

Wrist Flexion Contracture
If conservative treatment does not achieve sufficient extension, the wrist can be straightened by a carpal wedge osteotomy and thus brought into a better position for flexion strength of the fingers. In the carpal wedge osteotomy, a wedge is resected dorsally and radially from the carpus and the wrist area is straightened radially and dorsally. In preschool age, the osteosynthesis of the carpus is performed using transosseous PDS threads, in older children additionally with temporary K-wire fixation. In addition, a palmar forearm release is performed. The often thickened forearm fascia is cut, the wrist flexors are lengthened or cut in case of fibrotic remodeling. Dorsally, the proximal part of the ulnar wrist extensor is transposed to the distal part of the radial wrist extensor to strengthen the pull to the radial side. This operation brings the wrist into a functionally favorable middle position (Fig. 5.29) (Waters and Bae 2012).

5.3.4.3 Palm

Flexion Position of the Palm and Fingers 2-5
To improve the flexion position of both fingers 2–5 and the palm, a palmar release of fingers

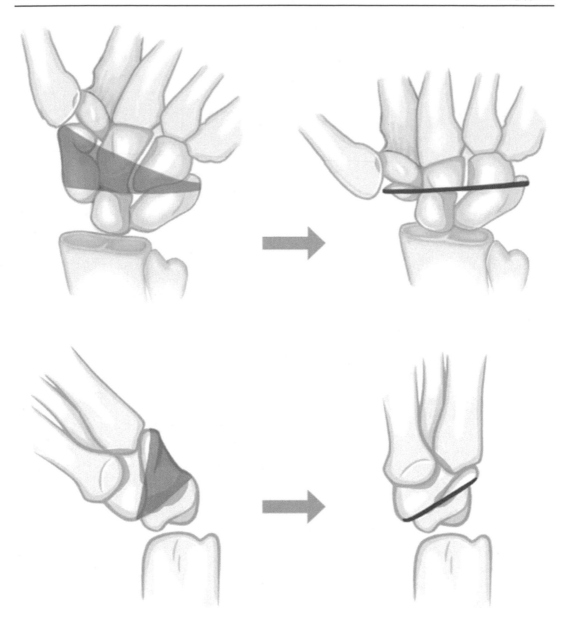

Fig. 5.29 Carpal wedge osteotomy. A dorsal wedge is resected from the carpus, straightening the wrist radially and dorsally. (© Children's Hospital Wilhelmstift, with kind permission)

2–5 by lengthening the skin in the palm may be useful.

5.3.4.4 Thumb

Thumb-in-Palm Deformity:
If the thumb cannot be released from the palm despite conservative treatment and there is also an adduction contracture, a surgical release is useful. All shortened structures are lengthened. Fibrous or tendinous parts of the M. interosseus or the M. adductor are cut, thus releasing the tension in the first intermetacarpal space (Fig. 5.30). Usually the thumb flexor tendon (FPL) is significantly shortened. It is lengthened by a Z-plasty at the level of the distal forearm

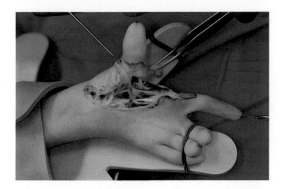

Fig. 5.30 Surgical release in a patient with a thumb-in-palm deformity. (© Children's Hospital Wilhelmstift, with kind permission)

and the base joint is temporarily fixed in a neutral position with a Kirschner wire. The skin in the area of the palmar thumb base joint and the palm is lengthened by grafts. The first interdigital fold is widened with a combined stretching flap from the back of the hand and an island flap from the index finger side.

5.4 Freeman-Sheldon Syndrome and Sheldon-Hall Syndrome

Freeman-Sheldon Syndrome
Freeman-Sheldon Syndrome (cranio-carpo-tarsal dysplasia, also known as Whistling-face Syndrome) is classified as a distal arthrogryposis. It is usually an autosomal dominant syndrome, but can also occur as a spontaneous mutation. This gene mutation causes changes in embryonic myosin, leading to muscle damage already in the womb.
Characteristics include:

- Microstomia: small "whistling" mouth and a flat-looking face,
- Ptosis: drooping eyelids/muscle weakness of the eyelid,
- Movement restrictions and malpositions of all joints of varying degrees.

The degree of physical disability varies greatly.

Sheldon-Hall Syndrome
Sheldon-Hall Syndrome is classified as a distal arthrogryposis and is considered a variant of Freeman-Sheldon Syndrome.
Characteristics include:

- Joint contractures of the hands,
- Joint contractures of the feet (pronounced talus verticalis, clubfoot),
- Facial abnormalities—a high palate and a small mouth opening (microstomia),
- Slanted eyelids, ptosis,
- Short stature.

The extent of physical disability varies greatly.

▶ The **myosin** is an essential component of the muscle and is involved in the conversion of energy into force and movement. It belongs to the motor proteins and is responsible for muscle contraction, among other things.

The hands of children with Freeman-Sheldon and Sheldon-Hall Syndrome show characteristic features that distinguish them from the "usual" forms of arthrogryposis:

- the wrist is in extension contracture and often shows ulnar deviation (Fig. 5.31b),
- the thumbs are tucked in (thumb-in-palm deformity) and can be rotated radially in the base joints (Fig. 5.31a), the palmar skin is often significantly shortened over the base joints, the end joints can show a radial deviation,
- a windblown hand deformity caused by an ulnar abduction of the finger base joints (Fig. 5.31b) exists in various degrees,
- the base and middle joints of the fingers as well as the end joints of the thumbs are often overstretched, indicating a lax palmar plate.

The malformation can vary greatly in severity.
From birth, treatment that strengthens the musculoskeletal system and improves

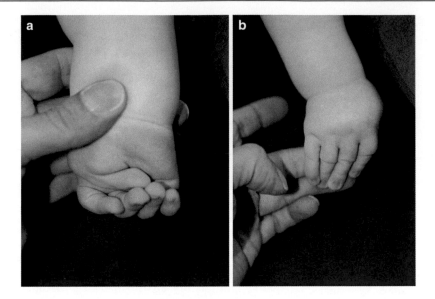

Fig. 5.31 a Right hand of a one-year-old boy with Sheldon-Hall Syndrome from the palmar side. The palm is significantly shortened, the fingers are in flexion and ulnar deviation. There is a severe thumb-in-palm deformity, the thumb is rotated in the base joint. The base and middle joints of the fingers as well as the thumb end joint are palmarly unstable and can be passively overstretched. **b** Right hand from the dorsal side shows the windblown hand deformity of the fingers. (© Children's Hospital Wilhelmstift, with kind permission)

contractures is important. Already in the first weeks of life, thermoplastic splints can support manual therapy and can be replaced by forearm orthoses with individual finger enclosure from about the sixth month of life.

5.4.1   Wrists

The **wrists** of children with Freeman-Sheldon or Sheldon-Hall Syndrome often show an extension contracture with existing ulnar deviation. The active and passive movement into flexion and radial abduction is limited. This insufficient mobility must be compensated by the elbow and shoulder joints, which are often also limited in their mobility. Early manual therapy to stretch the wrists into flexion and correct ulnar abduction can be supplemented by splint therapy already in infancy.

5.4.2   windblown hand deformity

In untreated windblown hand deformity, the progressive deviation of the fingers towards the ulnar side can lead to an overstretching of the radial collateral ligaments. The tendons do not pull centrally, which limits the strength of the fingers. Because of the ulnar deviation of the fingers, the opposition to the thumb becomes less efficient, weaker, and impossible with simultaneous thumb-in-palm deformity (Fig. 5.32a, b). Grasping is often only possible with both hands (Fig. 5.32c). So far, there is no evidence to support the benefits of permanent night splint treatment. However, our experience and reports from parents show that children are more skilled and have better strength after one year of treatment. During this time, the base joints have straightened towars the radial side and the lax ligaments have become noticeably more stable. Depending

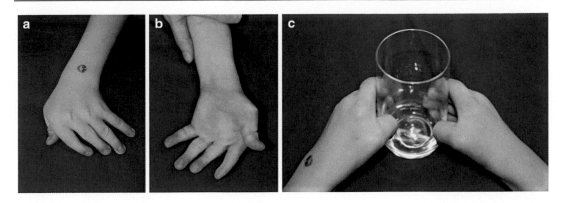

Fig. 5.32 a, b 6-year-old boy with Freeman-Sheldon syndrome at initial presentation. The wrist is in 20° extension and tends towards the ulnar side, the palm is shortened, the fingers are in a windblown hand deformity, the thumb is tucked into the palm and can neither be actively nor passively extended dorsally. The thumb end joints are hyperextended. The first interdigital fold is greatly narrowed. **c** Due to the deformities, a glass can only be held with both hands. (© Children's Hospital Wilhelmstift, with kind permission)

on the severity, night splint therapy may be required for several years. An early treatment phase in infancy and toddlerhood also has a positive effect on the child's motor and receptive skills.

5.4.3   Thumb-in-Palm Deformity

In Freeman-Sheldon and Sheldon-Hall syndrome, children exhibit similar anatomical changes to the thumb as in distal arthrogryposis. However, a thumb very tightly folded into the palm with pronounced adduction to the index finger is often found in addition, which only allows limited passive abduction as well as palmar and radialduction (Figs. 5.33a, 5.34a, b, 5.35a–c). In some cases, there may also be a rotation in the base joint towards the radial side. A significantly shortened palm intensifies the thumb-in-palm deformity.

Manual treatment and orthotic therapy are an important step in preparing for necessary thumb surgeries: the palm is expanded, the thumbs are partially led out of the thumb-in-palm deformity, and the position of the wrist in the splint is corrected. At the same time, the flexion contracture and the windblown hand deformity of the fingers are counteracted. Unstable base and middle joints of the fingers, which are often observed in

Freeman-Sheldon and Sheldon-Hall syndrome, are encased in a slight flexion of about 20°. This also applies to the thumb end joint.

5.5   Treatment Examples

5.5.1   Wrist extension contracture with ulnar deviation, shortened palm, thumb-in-palm and windblown hand deformity with unstable, lax proximal and middle joints of the fingers and the thumb's distal joint

Girl with Sheldon-Hall Syndrome. First presentation at the age of 8 months. Shoulder and elbow joints are well movable. The wrists are in 40° dorsal extension on both sides and can be passively corrected to 10° extension. Active flexion is not possible. The finger base joints are spontaneously in flexion, show a windblown hand deformity and cross over each other. The finger base and middle joints are unstable. The thumbs show a severe thumb-in-palm deformity. The base joints are not actively movable (Fig. 5.34a, b).

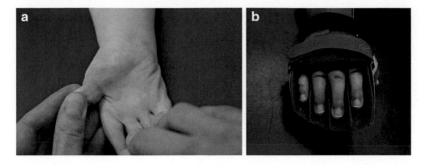

Fig. 5.33 a 22-month-old girl with Sheldon-Hall syndrome. The thumb can only be moved very slightly into palmar and radialduction. **b** The orthosis expands the palm, moves the thumb out of the palm, and corrects the windblown hand position of the fingers, while simultaneously splinting the wrist in flexion. A slight flexion of fingers 2-5 in the base and middle joints serves to stabilize the loosened palmar ligaments. (© Children's Hospital Wilhelmstift, with kind permission)

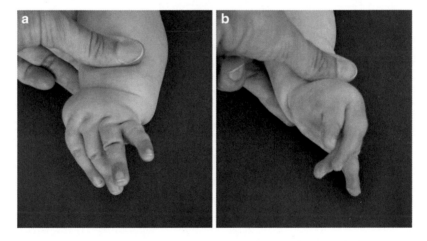

Fig. 5.34 a Left hand from the dorsal side. 8-month-old girl with Sheldon-Hall syndrome. The wrist is inclined towards the ulnar side and in extension contracture. The thumb is very tightly folded into the palm and cannot be moved actively. The base joints of fingers 2–5 lean strongly towards the ulnar side and the fingers overlap when moving. The base and middle joints of the fingers as well as the thumb end joint show instability of the palmar plate. The palm is shortened. **b** Left hand lateral view from radial side. (© Children's Hospital Wilhelmstift, with kind permission)

Manual treatments began in the first weeks of life, splint therapy from the first presentation at the age of 8 months. The splints were continuously adjusted during growth.

After 14 months of treatment, the girl can begin to actively move the thumbs out of the palm. The finger base joints are more stable. The wrists can now be actively moved from 40° extension to 20° extension and precision grips can be performed to some extent. For more powerful grips, better radial and palmar abduction of the thumbs and stabilization in the middle joints are necessary (Fig. 5.35a–c).

At the age of 3 years, surgical therapy is performed: Widening and deepening of the first interdigital fold using a combined rotation-expansion and island flap from the index finger. Detachment of the M. adductor pollicis at the distal portion of the 1st metacarpal, release of the M. adductor at the 3rd metacarpal. Extension

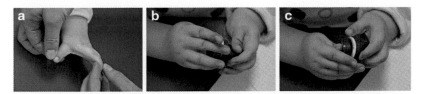

Fig. 5.35 a–c After 14 months of treatment, the thumb can be passively and actively led out of the palm to some extent. However, the severe soft tissue shortening at the level of the palmar thumb base joint does not allow for wide dorsal extension. The palm is widened, the base joints of the fingers are significantly straighter since they have been led out of ulnar deviation. The fingers no longer cross over each other. The finger base joints are somewhat more stable. (© Children's Hospital Wilhelmstift, with kind permission)

of the thumb flexor tendon by Z-plasty. Temporary thumb metacarpophalangeal joint arthrodesis and coverage of the remaining palmar skin defects with full-thickness skin grafts.

After removal of the K-wire 6 weeks postoperatively, the splint treatment was continued. Initially, the little patient received a thermoplastic forearm splint with thumb enclosure to counteract a tendency to reset due to scar traction (Fig. 5.27c). The fingers were left free, since wearing the splint for up to 20 hours per day was necessary and the use of the fingers for playing should remain possible. Six months later, a forearm orthosis with individual finger enclosure for all fingers was fitted for wearing at night (Fig. 5.33b).

At almost four years of age, both hands show better joint stability, the windblown hand deformity is only slightly noticeable. The wrists have a larger range of motion and can be actively flexed to 0°. The passive stretching of the right thumb into radial and palmar abduction is fully possible postoperatively. Overall, hand function and strength have significantly improved. The

girl is much more skillful. She can securely grasp larger objects with her right hand. Power grips have thus become possible and precision grips are more accurate (Fig. 5.36a–c).

Our recommendation at this time is to perform a surgical release of the opposite side, continue manual treatment, and wear night orthoses with individual finger enclosure to expand and improve grip functions and prevent recurrences.

5.5.2   Thumb-in-Palm Deformity

Boy with a thumb-in-palm deformity on both sides, more severe on the right than on the left side. First presentation at the age of 3 months (Fig. 5.37a, b). On this day, manual therapy and night-time splint treatment begin.

At the age of 12 months, active gripping has improved, but palmar and radial abduction are still incomplete. (Fig. 5.38a, b).

After 18 months of therapy, a therapy break is taken due to the positive result. One year

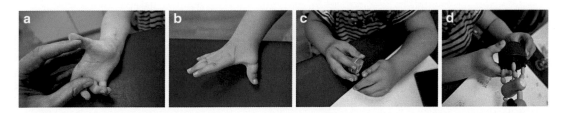

Fig. 5.36 a–d The same girl at the age of 3.9 years. After 3 years of conservative treatment and 9 months after surgical release of the right thumb. Passively, the thumb can be fully led into radial and palmarduction, actively this has improved significantly. The wrists have a larger range of motion and can be actively flexed to neutral position. The fingers only show a slight windblown hand deformity. The palm is fully expandable on both sides. All finger joints have stabilized and can be used more powerfully without hyperextension. (© Children's Hospital Wilhelmstift, with kind permission)

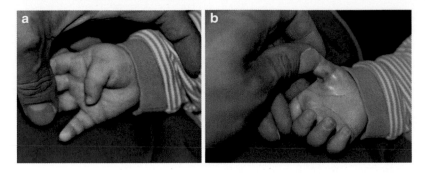

Fig. 5.37 **a** 3-month-old boy with a thumb-in-palm deformity. The thumb is folded into the palm and cannot be actively moved out of the palm. **b** During passive stretching, a clear palmar pull of the thenar muscles can be seen. The thumb only allows a slight passive movement. (© Children's Hospital Wilhelmstift, with kind permission)

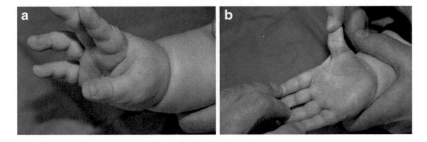

Fig. 5.38 **a** At the age of 12 months. After 9 months of manual therapy and splint treatment, the thumb can be actively moved out of the palm. **b** Passively, the thumb can be stretched further into palmar and radial abduction, the tension in the palm has decreased, the skin over the thumb base joint has stretched. (© Children's Hospital Wilhelmstift, with kind permission)

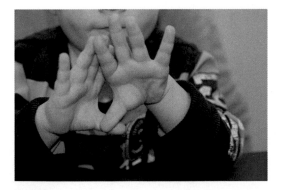

Fig. 5.39 At the age of three, after a one-year therapy break, the thumbs can be actively guided into a good, however still incomplete radial and palmar abduction. (© Children's Hospital Wilhelmstift, with kind permission)

later, at the age of three, the thumbs still show sufficient active palmar and radial abduction (Fig. 5.39).

At the age of five, the radial and palmar abduction of the right hand have worsened (Fig. 5.40a). Manual therapy is intensified and night-time splint treatment is resumed.

After 3 months, passive radial and palmar abduction is fully restored (Fig. 5.40b). Manual therapy and splint treatment are continued for another 6 months during this rapid growth phase.

Our recommendation during the entire growth period is:

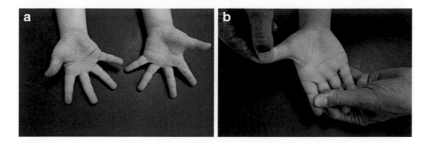

Fig. 5.40 a At the age of 5 years after a three-year therapy break. The right thumb pulls back into the palm. Therefore, splint treatment is resumed at night and manual therapy is intensified during the day. **b** Three months later at the follow-up control and splint adjustment. The right thumb can passively be fully (and actively largely) guided into palmar and radial abduction. In active movements, a slight adduction contracture is visible. (© Children's Hospital Wilhelmstift, with kind permission)

- manual stretching twice a day, e.g., before each tooth brushing.
- In a phase of accelerated growth, manual therapy can be supported by night-time splint treatment.

References

Agranovich O, Lakhina O (2020) ifssh ezine, Heft 40, Classification of upper limb deformities, S 11–15

Bahm J (2017) Bewegungsstörungen der oberen Extremität bei Kindern. Springer, Berlin

Kramer J, ten Velden M, Kafkes A, Basu S, Federico J, Kielhofner G (2021) COSA – Child occupational self assessment. User´s manual. (Version 2.2). The Board of Trustees of the University of Illinois. Schulz-Kirchner Verlag – Idstein, Deutschland

Kraus E, Romein E (2015) Pädiatrisch Ergotherapeutisches Assessment und Prozessinstrument (PEAP). Schulz-Kirchner Verlag GmbH, Idstein

Mundlos S, Horn D (2014) Limb malformations/An atlas of genetic disorders of limb development. Springer, Berlin

Waters PM, Bae DS (2012) Pediatric hand and upper limb surgery: a practical guide. Lippincott Williams and Wikens, United States

The Scar

6

Contents

The scar is a collagen-fiber-rich, cell and vessel-poor connective tissue that replaces local tissue in case of skin injuries or after substantial tissue loss. This collagenous connective tissue is less elastic than the connective tissue of healthy skin. If it extends into deeper tissue layers, adhesions can form between tissue layers such as tendons, capsules, and ligaments. These adhesions can cause pain and restrict mobility, especially if the scar crosses a joint.

Scars are initially numb, as the smallest skin nerves are severed during operations or injuries. During the healing process, they can become hypersensitive. A scar is initially red and fades over the course of scar maturation, until it is usually lighter than the surrounding skin. Exceptions exist in people with dark skin or after intense sunbathing, which is why strong sunlight should be avoided on the scar tissue throughout the entire scar maturation process.

From the day of the injury until complete maturation, a scar goes through several maturation phases. Scar maturation lasts about 1 to 2 years, two years especially for large wound defects, such as after burns. Age has a significant influence on scar formation. Wound healing is very good in the first year of life and deteriorates until puberty. During puberty, it is negatively influenced by hormones. In children up to about the seventh year of life, the formation of adhesions is less intense, so fewer movement restrictions remain due to connective tissue crosslinks. In the first years of life, children do not go easy on themselves, which is why a longer period of immobilization is usually required after injuries or operations than in adolescents or adults. Movement exercises and scar treatment can often only begin later. One might suspect that this promotes the formation of adhesions. However, children compensate for this by using their hand much faster and in a more automated way in everyday life.

Other influences on scar formation include:

- The skin type: the darker the skin, the more often hypertrophies occur.

- The type of injury: lacerations, contused wounds, surgical wounds, burns, etc.
- The location: scars on the shoulder or sternum are more prone to hypertrophies, scars over flexion creases more often cause movement restrictions.
- Genetic predisposition and
- Wound hygiene.

6.1   Scar Phases

In the literature, **scar phases** are described differently. Generally, healing, regardless of the origin of a wound, proceeds in maturation phases that overlap or merge into each other. The maturation phases described below refer to uncomplicated wound healing, e.g., after a surgical elective procedure. In the case of wound infections, lacerations, and contused wounds, the wound healing phases are extended.

Scar Maturation Phases

- Exudative Phase
- Proliferation Phase
- Reparative Phase
- Remodeling Phase

(Waldner-Nilsson 2013a, b).

Timeline of Wound Healing Processes
1. Vascular reaction approx. 0–3 days
2. Blood clotting approx. 0–1 day
3. Inflammation approx. 0–14 days
4. Tissue regeneration approx. 1–25 days
5. Epithelialization approx. 1–12 days
6. Contraction approx. 3–20 days
7. Scar transformation approx. 9–24 months

(Waldner-Nilsson 2013a, b; Asmussen and Söllner 1993).

6.1.1   Exudative Phase

The exudative phase, which begins immediately after surgery, includes the vascular reaction,

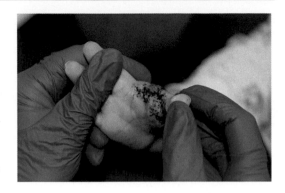

Fig. 6.1 First interdigital fold 6 days after pollicization (Chap. 3). The wound is closed, but still vulnerable, red, and swollen. (© Children's Hospital Wilhelmstift, with kind permission)

blood clotting, and inflammation. Blood clotting and vasoconstriction (= vessel contraction) begin postoperatively within seconds and stop further blood loss. A few minutes after wound closure, vasodilation (= physiological reaction for better blood circulation) begins. This leads to a wound edema and typical signs of inflammation such as redness, heat, swelling, pain, and functional impairment occur (Fig. 6.1). The acute inflammatory phase lasts 4–6 days, after which the signs of inflammation slowly subside. Contaminations, infections, insufficient rest, and intensive movement therapy starting too early prolong the inflammation phase and induce increased scar formation. The low resilience of the tissue must be taken into account during this phase. Early functional scar mobilization directly on the scar should only begin at the end of the exudative phase. The production of type 3 collagen begins.

6.1.2   Proliferative Phase

The proliferative phase already begins parallel to the exudative phase. During the proliferative phase, epithelialization as well as tissue and connective tissue regeneration occur. Necrotic tissue at the wound edge is broken down, cell- and vessel-rich granulation tissue forms (Fig. 6.2). This wound healing phase begins approximately from the 2nd to 5th day after

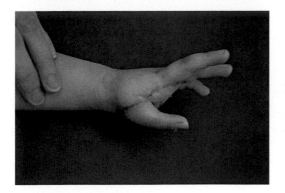

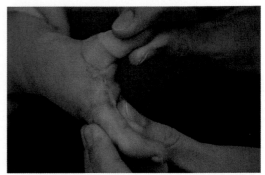

Fig. 6.2 First interdigital fold three weeks after pollicization. The scar is red and hardened, the swelling is subsiding, the wound is firmly closed. (© Children's Hospital Wilhelmstift, with kind permission)

Fig. 6.3 First interdigital fold six weeks after pollicization. The swelling is further subsiding, the scar is slightly sunken and strongly hardened. (© Children's Hospital Wilhelmstift, with kind permission)

injury and lasts until about the 21st to 25th day. The production of type 3 collagen continues and is supplemented by the connection of type 1 and 2 collagen. Fibroblasts are able to add type 3 collagen fibers in the direction of function due to functional mechanical stimuli. This creates the basis for later tissue function. The suture removal takes place during this time, i.e., 10 to 12 days postoperatively. Remnants of self-dissolving sutures can be wiped off 3–6 weeks postoperatively.

6.1.3   Reparative Phase

The reparative phase begins from the 3rd to 5th day after surgery. In the granulation tissue, the first collagen fibers form, which continue to densify postoperatively and increase the tear resistance of the wound. Three weeks postoperatively, approximately 15% of the final firmness is achieved (Madden 1990) and after 6 weeks approximately 50% (Westaby 1985) (Fig. 6.3). The pressure and tensile-load capacity increases due to the formed crosslinks. Adhesions always occur during the scar maturation phases. The aim is to minimize their restrictive effects on the range of motion. Passive stretching and active function-specific techniques are particularly suitable for this.

6.1.4   Remodeling Phase

The synthesis and lysis of collagen lasts approximately 9–12 months, and for large wounds, up to two years. The collagen fibers begin to align themselves in parallel (Fig. 6.4). They stabilize and gain firmness, the immature type 3 collagen transforms into mature type 1 collagen. At the end of wound healing, the proportion of collagen type 3 to type 1 is 10%, which is similar to normal skin. Since no elastin is formed, flexibility is lacking compared

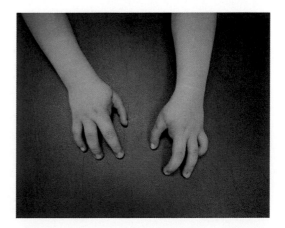

Fig. 6.4 Comparison of scar formation after bilateral pollicization. Left hand 15 months postoperatively, right hand 7 months postoperatively. The older scar is lighter and less retracted. (© Children's Hospital Wilhelmstift, with kind permission)

to healthy skin. As long as the scar has a reddened appearance, the transformation is not yet complete.

6.2 Scar Treatment

The goal of **scar treatment** is a functional and aesthetic scar as well as good mobility of the tissue layers, without destroying the newly formed tissue.

At the beginning of the treatment, infections must be ruled out and the appearance and trophicity of the scar must be assessed for: firmness and maturity, atrophy or hypertrophy, keloids, severe swelling, contractures, circulatory disorders, and adhesions. Restrictions of joint mobility due to existing adhesions become apparent in passive and active movements. During the healing process, hyper- and hyposensitivity are checked by touching and pressing on the scar.

Scar massages are often uncomfortable at first. Especially in small children, it is therefore important to find an appropriate dosage. The therapist must build a basic trust in the child in order to be able to carry out the scar massage successfully and consistently and to slowly approach the scar treatment. Children often react with defense and emotional outbursts. An increase in the intensity of the scar massage can usually occur from the third postoperative week. Then adhesions can be dissolved by directly moving the tissue layers.

After the immobilization has ended, children move the affected hand early on their own, which contributes to active scar mobilization in everyday life. However, this does not replace passive manual scar treatment.

Caution:
A scar can only be therapeutically influenced during the maturation phase. Once the scar is mature, it can only be altered by surgical intervention or laser treatment followed by conservative therapy.

6.2.1 Immediately After the Operation

Immediately after the operation, the treatment should be carried out depending on the diagnosis and age of the patient or after consultation with the operating or treating doctor. Light fascial shifts outside the direct scar area should be achieved. This should be done without strong pressure and without cream with gloves at a sterile workplace.

The mobilization stimulates the scar tissue to align longitudinally and the scar becomes more elastic as a result. An important part of the treatment are decongestant measures and lymph-activating techniques from distal to proximal for edema reduction. After tenolysis (surgical loosening of adhered tendons), it is important to start with gentle passive and active mobilization of the joints from the first postoperative day to counteract new adhesions.

6.2.2 Approx. from the 14th postoperative day

Approx. from the 14th postoperative day after suture removal, the treatment is carried out by:

- Hand baths: they clean the skin and support the removal of old skin.
- Regular moisturizing and massaging of the scar is necessary to make it supple and prevent adhesions. The scar tissue does not produce its own fat, therefore treatment with a rich cream is necessary, which together with the scar massage takes place at least $3\times$ daily. It is not proven that expensive scar creams have a positive effect on scar maturation.
- Depending on the injury, if possible, passive and active movements of the joints to avoid contractures.

Depending on the operation, clinical picture, and scar condition, close checks are carried out. Passive and active mobilization as well as manual therapeutic treatment is intensified and, if necessary, aid therapy is started. A gentle, pain-free scar massage is begun. For scars crossing joints, early mobilization is beneficial to counteract adhesions and contractures. Since small children resist being held and show a strong emotional reaction, careful observation and adjustment of the dosage are very important. The scars are massaged in both directions, both from distal to proximal and from proximal to distal, with light circular movements lateral to the scar. In this phase, therapeutic intervention is particularly important, as a functional arrangement can only take place if the necessary stimuli occur. Stimuli that are too strong can lead to increased proliferation and thus cause hypertrophic scars. Stretching or compression should therefore always be dosed below the pain threshold.

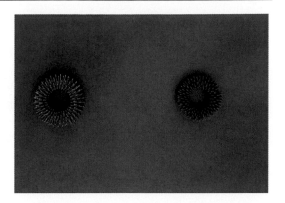

Fig. 6.5 Arthro rings in two different sizes. (© Children's Hospital Wilhelmstift, with kind permission)

6.2.3 From the 21st postoperative day

The treatment **from the 21st postoperative day** in the event of an uncomplicated course: An intensive scar massage is started. Cross-friction (massage technique for shifting between superficial scar and deep tissue layers) is also used to dissolve adhesions, for which scar sticks, cupping glasses (Fig. 6.6) and tapes (Fig. 6.17) are suitable. For small children, treatment with the finger is recommended, as the therapist is most sensitive this way. The scar is worked from distal to proximal and from proximal to distal. With stronger pressure, the scar tissue is shifted laterally. The scar massage can, if postoperatively allowed, be intensified by pre-stretching. These techniques are painful. To increase tolerance, parents must distract their children well. Only in this way is intensive treatment possible. A heat treatment before the scar massage is helpful to make the tissue more stretchable and supple. Now a desensitization of the scar tissue is indicated, by gentle stimuli with soft brushes. In the course, the therapist can intensify the sensory stimuli through vibration, spiky massage balls and arthro rings (Fig. 6.5). Other possibilities for desensitization are warm and cold cherry stone, rapeseed and pebble baths, playing in the sand, kneading dough, etc.

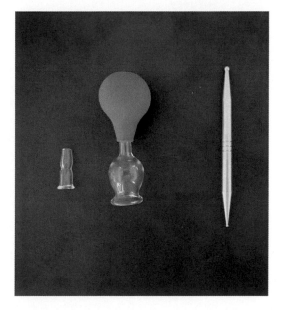

Fig. 6.6 Cupping glass with two attachments and a scar stick. (© Children's Hospital Wilhelmstift, with kind permission)

Desensitization is important so that the hand is not only used well, but the child can also tolerate and process tactile stimuli (Chap. 1).

Desensitization includes three components:

- Touching different materials,
- Manipulating/moving different materials,
- Vibration at different frequencies.

(Waldner-Nilsson 2013a, b).

6.2.4   Remodeling phase

In the remodeling phase, the scar treatment should continue with strong pressure and intensive stimuli on the tissue. Through consistent scar treatment, the elasticity and resilience of the tissue can significantly improve. The parents massage and grease the scar at least until half a year after surgery. An improvement in functionality as well as cosmetics is possible up to two years after the operation.

6.2.5   Scar treatment after free flap surgery

Free flap surgeries are used for defect coverage in extensive tissue damage. The removal is done including the veins and arteries, which are microsurgically connected to the local vascular system. The therapeutic approach after skin grafts and free flap surgeries must be coordinated with the surgeon, as different procedures are used:

- The transplanted split or full-thickness skin needs about 3 weeks to grow onto the subcutaneous tissue, which is why gentle scar mobilization is only carried out after this time.
- The removal site of the graft is included in the scar treatment.
- To prevent contractures in joint-crossing transplant scars, early functional passive and active follow-up treatment must be carried out.
- Provision with compression, silicone as well as splints is indicated earlier in grafts.

▶ In addition to the general scar treatment described here, special follow-up treatments are discussed in the respective chapters.

6.3   Complications

Complications must be detected early and treated promptly. These include:

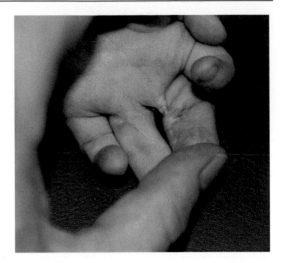

Fig. 6.7 One year after syndactyly separation. The scar contracture prevents the extension of the middle finger. The scar is fully mature, therefore scar excision is necessary. This is followed by early therapeutic aftercare to prevent recurrence. (© Children's Hospital Wilhelmstift, with kind permission)

- Scar contractures,
- Atrophic scars,
- Keloids,
- Hypertrophic scars

In addition, there may be hyper- or hyposensitivity.

6.3.1   Scar Contractures

Scar contractures are scars that have shrunk, are inelastic, and hard. They contract like a band. If they cross a joint, they can lead to severe movement restrictions (Fig. 6.7).

6.3.2   Atrophic Scars

Atrophic scars are sunken scars. They often form after inflammation due to damage to the corium (dermis). Scars are below the skin level. Acne and chickenpox scars are typical atrophic scars.

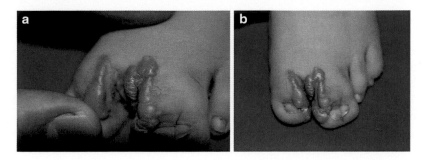

Fig. 6.8 a, b Three months after syndactyly separation. Keloids are raised, bulging, not delimited, and grow beyond the original scar borders. (© Children's Hospital Wilhelmstift, with kind permission)

6.3.3   Keloids

Keloids are also called hypertrophic scars or connective tissue proliferations. These scars grow excessively beyond the actual wound edges. They itch, are hypersensitive, burn, and are often also painful (Fig. 6.8a, b). The risk of keloid formation increases with increasing skin pigmentation, and there is a genetic predisposition.

6.3.4   Hypertrophic Scars

Hypertrophic scars are raised, but unlike keloids, they do not exceed the original scar area. Hypertrophies often form when scars run over tension lines or joints, with large scars or secondary healing (Fig. 6.9). They occur more frequently 6 months after trauma and, unlike keloids, are easy to treat.

6.3.5   Procedures for Scar Complications

Conservative treatment is sometimes insufficient for severe hypertrophic scars and keloids. In addition, the following procedures may be necessary:

- Glucocorticosteroids,
- Cryosurgery,
- Surgical techniques,

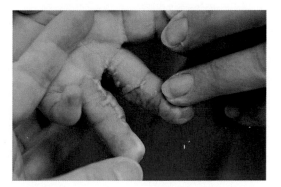

Fig. 6.9   Five months after syndactyly separation. The hypertrophic scars protrude above the skin level but are well delimited. The hypertrophic scars pull the middle and ring fingers into a deviation and flexion contracture. (© Children's Hospital Wilhelmstift, with kind permission)

- Laser treatment,
- Microneedling (contraindicated in keloids),
- Radiation therapy.

6.4   Aids for Scar Treatment

During the maturation process of scars and in case of complications, various aids can support healing in addition to intensive manual treatment. They are used individually depending on the degree of maturation and complication:

- Silicone,
- Compression bandages,
- Splints/orthoses,
- Tapes.

6.4.1   Silicone

When scars are significantly hypertrophic and/
or restrict movement, the use of silicone is beneficial. Silicone pads make scars more elastic,
smoother, and softer. This facilitates subsequent
manual treatment, as deeper layers of tissue can
be massaged and adhesions can be better loosened. Depending on the nature and location of
the scar, various silicone products are selected:

- Silicone patches,
- Silicone finger cots,
- RTV silicone putty,
- HTV silicone pads,
- Silon-Tex,
- Silicone gel.

▶   The complete air seal of the
skin by the silicone increases the local
skin temperature and retains moisture
in place. This inhibits the formation of
fibroblasts and influences collagen formation. The scars become softer, more
elastic, and flatter.

Caution:
Silicone should only be used after complete wound healing, as the skin is sof-
tened by the silicone. Small skin defects
cannot close under silicone or will even
enlarge. Due to the air seal, the silicone
should not remain on the skin for more
than 14 hours. In case of skin diseases,
such as neurodermatitis, silicone treatment is contraindicated. Before silicone
treatment, the skin must be cleaned with
removal of dirt, sweat, and cream resi-
dues. The silicone itself must be cleaned
with liquid soap and water after each use
and laid on a foil to dry. This prevents
skin irritations and allergic reactions. The
hygiene measures enable a long silicone
therapy.

6.4.1.1   Silicone Patches
Silicone patches come in varying thickness and
elasticity. The scar treatment on hands and fingers of toddlers requires thin and elastic patches.
The patch is cut to the shape of the scar and
stuck directly onto the cleaned skin with the
adhesive side. In small children, the patch can
be fixed with a self-adhesive bandage. The patch
unfolds its full effect when worn under a compression glove. It can be removed very easily
and painlessly from the skin. When removing
the patch, care must be taken not to damage or
stick it together. With good care, it can be used
for several weeks (Fig. 6.10a, b). If small parti-
cles peel off the patch and the adhesive power
decreases, it should be replaced.

6.4.1.2   Silicone/Gel Finger Cot
The **silicone/gel finger cot** is a combination
of silicone/gel and compression (Fig. 6.11a).
Pressure on the scar reduces swelling and keeps
the scar at skin level. It is particularly suitable for
treating the finger stump after distal amputation.
The silicone/gel keeps the scars supple, the compression shapes the stump. It is important that the
finger cot fits very tightly at the tip and that no air
cushion forms between the finger cot and the skin
(Fig. 6.11b). After about ten minutes of wearing,
small grooves of the finger cot must be visible on
the skin. If this is not the case, the compression
is too weak and a smaller size must be chosen
or a custom-made compression glove must be
used. Due to the silicone/gel, the wearing time is
no longer than 14 hours per day. The finger cot
is cleaned daily. For this, it is turned inside out.
There are also finger cots for scar compression
without silicone/gel; under these silicone gel can
be applied to the scar, if necessary.

6.4.1.3   RTV Silicone Putty
RTV silicone putty (= room temperature vulcanizing silicone putty) consists of two components that are processed into a mass by
kneading. At room temperature, the mass
hardens after about 2 minutes and remains
in the desired shape in a slightly elastic state

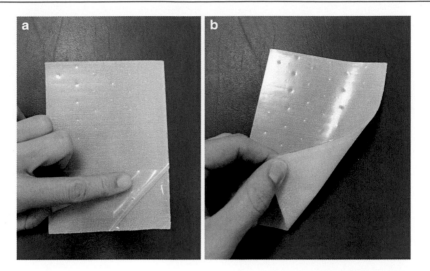

Fig. 6.10 a, b The silicone patch for toddlers' hands must be thin and elastic to optimally lay it around joints and in between finger folds. (© Children's Hospital Wilhelmstift, with kind permission)

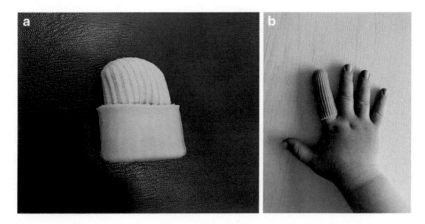

Fig. 6.11 a, b Silicone/gel finger cot: the silicone/gel keeps the skin supple, warm, and moist, and the compression exerts pressure on the scar. These ready-made finger cots fit depending on the finger, age, and size of the child from the 4th to 8th year of life. (© Children's Hospital Wilhelmstift, with kind permission)

(Fig. 6.12a). This two-component silicone is well suited as a pad or as an impression for an HTV silicone pad. If the two-component silicone is used as a pad, the material should not be applied too thickly, as it will then become too heavy. It lasts about 4–6 weeks until it loses its structure with daily use. The silicone can be worn under a splint or a compression glove or attached with a self-adhesive bandage. If a thermoplastic splint is modeled over such a pad, this combination must be readjusted after 4–6 weeks (Fig. 6.12b). The thermoplastic splint must always be modeled on the previously made pad, as the two-component silicone is quite thick and thus changes the shape of the splints.

6.4.1.4 HTV Silicone Pads

HTV silicone pads (= high-temperature vulcanizing silicone) are particularly useful for concave structures, such as the palms or interdigital

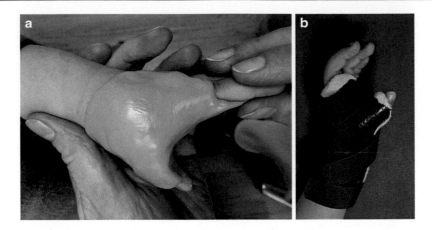

Fig. 6.12 **a** The silicone putty is modeled into the first interdigital fold. This imprint is used to make an HTV silicone pad. **b** However, it can also be worn much more thinly under a thermoplastic splint. (© Kinderkrankenhaus Wilhelmstift, with kind permission)

folds (Fig. 6.13a and 6.14a–c). The pads can be used in combination with splints or compression stockings to treat scars, to widen interdigital folds (Fig. 6.13a, b), or to perform position corrections (Fig. 6.14b, c). The production is complex and time-consuming. It is carried out by a medical supply store according to an imprint with two-component silicone or plaster. The material is light, easy to clean, and durable. It is recommended to let the edges taper off thinly. Due to its thin nature, it fits under compression gloves and splints.

> **Caution:**
> Only silicones for medical use should be used.

6.4.1.5 Silon-Tex©

Silon-Tex© is a textile carrier material onto which a medical silicone is applied. It is used for active scars and is individually sewn into the compression gloves (Fig. 6.15a, b). It can be used very well for scars on fingers or the back of the hand. Due to the fixation in the glove, it is very suitable

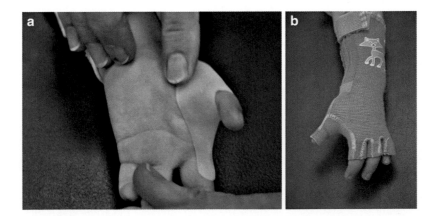

Fig. 6.13 **a, b** Three months after pollicization. The HTV pad improves the scar with its silicone component and widens the first interdigital fold. It keeps the thumb in abduction and opposition. It is worn in combination with a compression glove that presses the pad tightly against the skin. (© Kinderkrankenhaus Wilhelmstift, with kind permission)

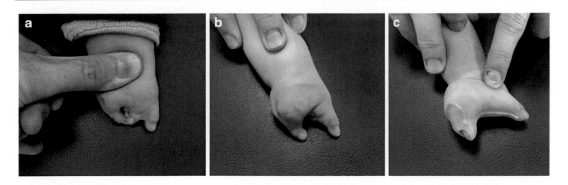

Fig. 6.14 **a** 9-month-old girl with symbrachydactyly-like changes of the right hand. The right hand has a short hypoplastic thumb, a small finger, and three end members of fingers 2–4. **b** 10 weeks after surgical resection of fingers 2–4 and rotation expansion flap. **c** The silicone pad with metal reinforcement both treats the scar and stretches the little finger into an upright position. A compression glove is worn over the pad. (© Kinderkrankenhaus Wilhelmstift, with kind permission)

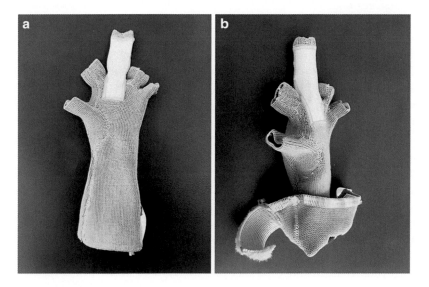

Fig. 6.15 **a, b** Compression glove with sewn-in Silon-Tex on the middle finger, turned inside out. (© Children's Hospital Wilhelmstift, with kind permission)

for toddlers, as slipping of the silicone is avoided. The Silon-Tex must not encircle the finger or hand, as this would impair blood circulation. This material is not suitable for scars that run concavely, such as in the palm of the hand or in the interdigital folds. Here, a silicone pad is needed to ensure skin contact of the silicone.

Caution:
Silon-Tex must not encircle a finger or hand, otherwise there is a risk of circulatory disruption. For compression gloves, cooperation with an experienced medical supply store is necessary.

6.4.1.6 Silicone Gel

Silicone gel is a gel that forms a film on the skin, similar to a spray plaster. The silicone is not suitable for scar massage, it should be applied to clean skin after the massage.

> **Caution:**
> In small children, silicone gel should only be used if the gel cannot be licked off or rubbed into the eyes, e.g. under a splint or a compression glove.

6.4.2   Compression Bandages

6.4.2.1 Silicone/Gel Finger Cot

See 6.4.1.2.

6.4.2.2 Custom Compression Gloves

For small children with altered anatomy due to malformations, a **custom compression glove** is suitable. To achieve optimal compression pressure, the child's hand must be measured with slight tension at skin level (Chap. 4). A sewn-on zipper makes it easier to put on the glove (Fig. 6.13b and 6.16c). The recommended wearing time in scar therapy is 23 hours. The constant pressure exerted by the compression on the scar tissue prevents the formation of excess scar tissue or treats it, if already present. The compression pressure arranges the collagen tissue parallel to the skin surface. The scar becomes more supple, flexible, and its thickness decreases. Additionally, the pressure relieves pain and itching. When silicone products are used at the same time, they are pressed tightly against the skin by the compression and can thus fully unfold their effect. The compression glove is cleaned by hand washing or in the washing machine at a maximum of 40° Celsius with detergent without fabric softener, even with sewn-in Silon-Tex (Fig. 6.15a, b). An additional glove is especially appropriate with a permanent wearing time. A glove with Silion-Tex must be taken off after a maximum of 14 hours and a change to a compression stocking without Silon-Tex must be made.

6.4.2.3 Interim Gloves

An **interim glove** is a ready-made glove that is offered in various sizes for teenagers and adults. Depending on the manufacturer, the gloves can be shortened in length both at the fingers and at the forearm without damaging the material. Their durability is 6–8 weeks. Therefore, they are a good transitional solution for treating severe swelling until a custom supply is sensible.

6.4.3   Thermoplastic Splints and Orthoses

6.4.3.1 Thermoplastic Splints

Thermoplastic splints for scar treatment are primarily used when the scars are located in the palm or run in interdigital folds (Fig. 6.12b).

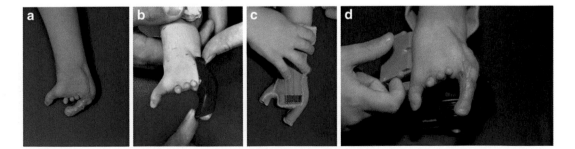

Fig. 6.16   a–c After toe transplantation to build up the little finger side in monodactylous symbrachydactyly with scar-related radial malposition. This glove splint was made to treat the scar and straighten the finger from its malposition. **d** After just two days of treatment, the finger position has significantly improved, the scar is flatter. The treatment was continued for another 4 months. (© Children's Hospital Wilhelmstift, with kind permission)

These scars tend to pull the fingers into flexion or the thumb into adduction. The splints are made after wound healing, swelling reduction, or K-wire removal. Their task is to stretch the skin and the deeper-lying scars and to maintain the stretch for several hours each day. This stimulates the scar tissue to align longitudinally and become more elastic and stretchable. Contractures are thus avoided.

6.4.3.2 Orthoses with Individual Finger Enclosure

For the simultaneous treatment of several fingers, **orthoses with individual finger enclosure** are needed (Chap. 2, 4, 5 and 8). The scars are kept under tension by the orthosis, which counteracts contractures.

6.4.3.3 Glove-Splint

The **Glove-Splint** (Chap. 4) can be used for scar and contracture treatment. The skin measurements for the glove are taken with slight tension to achieve sufficient compression. The small thermoplastic splint (Fig. 6.16b), which brings the finger into the desired position, is placed into the sewn-on pocket (Fig. 6.16c) (Chap. 4). Silicone gel is used for additional silicone treatment.

6.4.3.4 Dynamic Quengel Splints

To stretch the scar several times a day, a **dynamic Quengel splint** or a dynamic extension or flexion orthosis (Chap. 8) can be used. Through a small spring joint, the affected joint is stretched into the desired position and kept under tension. These splints are worn several times a day for a maximum of 30 minutes. Longer application (more than 30 minutes at a time) can impair circulation.

6.4.4 Kinesio or Crosstapes

Kinesio- or Crosstapes are also suitable for scar treatment (Fig. 6.17). They are applied to the area of the scar from the remodeling phase onwards.

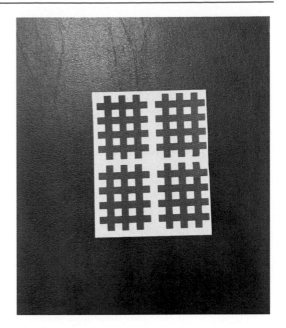

Fig. 6.17 Medium-sized Crosstape for sticking on scars to loosen superficial adhesions. (© Children's Hospital Wilhelmstift, with kind permission)

They cause tension or friction on the skin when moving. This can loosen slight adhesions.

6.5 Summary

The treatment of scars significantly contributes to better mobility after surgery. It is important to communicate this to parents, even if the children refuse and the scar massage is very uncomfortable or painful. With regular treatment, sensitivity decreases and pain subsides quickly. Through routine and distraction strategies, children usually engage in therapy. Initially, pain medication before treatment may be useful. In these cases, consultation with the treating physician should be held, as well as in cases of uncertainty in aftercare.

References

Asmussen PD, Söllner B (1993) Prinzipien der Wundheilung, Bd 1. Hippokrates, Stuttgart

Madden JW (1990) Wound healing: the biological basis of hand surgery. In: Hunter JM, Schneider LH, Mackin EJ, Callahan AD (Hrsg) Rehabilitation of the hand, 3. Aufl. Mosby, St. Louis

Waldner-Nilsson B (2013a) Handrehabilitation Band 1 Verletzungen. Springer, Heidelberg

Waldner-Nilsson B (2013b) Handrehabilitation Band 2 Verletzungen. Springer, Heidelberg

Westaby S (1985) Fundamentals of wound healing. In: Westabi S (Hrsg) Wound care. Heinemann Medical Books, London

Aid Provision

7

Contents

In patients with malformations, a therapeutic holistic functional analysis (based on the ICF) and a consultation on aids by occupational therapists and/or specialists from a medical supply store should take place at regular intervals appropriate to the age. Various assessments can be used for this. An annual review is desirable for severely affected children.

A rough distinction is made between aids and adaptations. Both are intended to promote or support the child's ability to act. This is especially necessary when pain and/or rapid fatigue occur, a new activity is being learned, or for performing tasks at work.

In children with dysmelia, prefabricated aids often cannot be used. In order to manufacture custom adaptations or aids, cooperation with a medical supply store is necessary.

7.1 Body Hygiene/Dressing and Undressing

- Handle extension for toilet hygiene, hairbrush, shower sponge
- Shower toilet/toilet seat with backrest, armrest and leg stool
- Shower chair/bath lounger
- Sliding boards
- Built-up handle for toothbrush
- Nail clippers with suction cups
- Button aid
- Rubber shoelaces
- Dressing tree
- Sock aid
- Tube key/tube emptier e.g. for toothpaste
- Extension of the faucet handle
- Handle on walls

7.2 Eating and Drinking

- Protractor
- One-handed board/board with attached knife
- Cutting aid
- Bottle opener
- Electric lid opener
- Peeler (finger peeler)
- Angled cutlery/cutlery with loops (Fig. 7.1a–c)
- Anti-slip film
- Plate with raised edge
- Feeding cup/cup with handle
- Helparm
- Apple cutter
- Dish brush with suction cups for washing up
- Footstool

7.3 School/Hobby

- Pencil aids (Fig. 7.2)
- Thick pencils
- Anti-slip foil
- Helparm
- Ruler with weight
- One-handed scissors with suction cups/ Scissors with spring etc.
- Computer/Laptop systems
- Ergonomic computer mouse
- Electronically height-adjustable tables and chairs
- Gripper
- Card holder

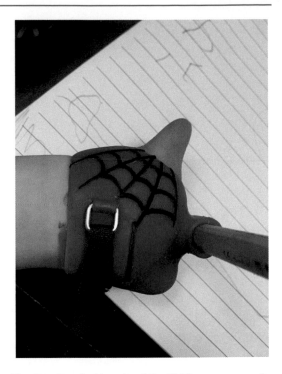

Fig. 7.2 Pencil aid made of Streifi-Flex to measure for the care of a child with dysmelia. The pencil is clamped into a silicone shaft. Pencil guidance is now possible for the child through arm movement. (© Stolle Sanitätshaus Hamburg, with kind permission)

- Seat with table and supported feet
- Physioform wedge, for example for the lateral position

In school or at home at the dining table or desk, a workplace analysis should always be carried out for children with malformations. Even

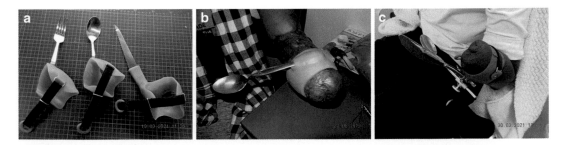

Fig. 7.1 **a** Custom cutlery aids made of Streifi-Flex with thumb hole, rings are attached to the Velcro straps as closure aids. **b** Cutlery aid made of Streifi-Flex to measure, as stump supply after traumatic amputation of the hand and wrist **c** Combination cutlery aid made of Streifi-Flex to measure as stump supply in dysmelia. (© Stolle Sanitätshaus Hamburg, with kind permission)

problems caused by instability in the MP joint can be reduced by a good seating adjustment.

Good sitting position = better trunk stability = better support of the forearm and thus better holding of the pencil.

The same applies to any activity at the table, such as eating: the more stable the child sits, the more freely it can operate the cutlery. Good foot support is always important to ensure an upright position of the trunk.

7.4   Locomotion

- Various wheelchairs
- Walker
- Rollators
- Leg orthoses
- Rehab stroller with footrest
- Standing trainer

For example, when sitting, a distinction is made between passive and active sitting for severely affected AMC children. Should the child have a stable trunk to be able to act freely with the hands, or should the child actively participate in the stability in the trunk? Foot support is important for both types of sitting.

7.5   Orthotic Care Upper Extremity

- Orthoses for stabilizing the proximal joints with active mobility of the distal joints, for example, the erection of the wrist with free finger mobility for everyday life
- Night splints for contracture prophylaxis
- Orthoses with a joint for static-progressive stretching of the wrists and fingers
- Orthoses for raising the thumb from the palm
- Nerve replacement splint
- Aids for performing replacement grips
- Steering wheel aids (Fig. 7.3a–c)

7.6   Other Aids

- Door handle extensions
- Window handle extensions
- Support pillows
- Nursing pillows

Aid provision should always take place through an interdisciplinary team. Usually, a recommendation for an aid is first made by therapists/educators/ parents or other professionals who work with the child. The pediatrician or orthopedist prescribes the necessary aids. With the prescription, a medical

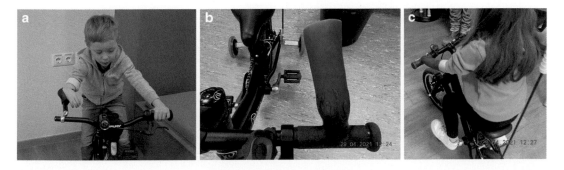

Fig. 7.3   a Steering wheel aid for the right hand in the case of a non-surgically treated RLD on the right. In addition to guiding the steering wheel, this compensates for the shortened arm and the resulting shoulder and spinal column malposition during cycling. **b** Custom-made steering wheel aid made of Streifi-Flex for the left hand in case of dysmelia. The shaft construction ensures a compensation of the length difference and a quick pulling out of the stump in case of fall. The shortening of the arm is compensated. **c** First driving attempts with the new steering wheel aid. This should be accompanied and practiced in a therapeutic setting. (© Stolle Sanitätshaus Hamburg, with kind permission)

supply store is visited, which carries out the provision. The medical supply store takes care of, among other things, forwarding the cost estimate to the health insurance company. Often, the approval of the aid takes weeks or months, so that the needs of the child change again in the meantime. If the health insurance company rejects the aid, a written objection should definitely be submitted.

Upon delivery of the aid, the adjustment and instruction must always be carried out by the medical supply store. Handling the aid is a therapeutic intervention and must be practiced during treatment with the patient. A review and adjustment is regularly carried out during the child's growth and development.

Materials, Manufacturing Types, Tips, Tricks

8

Contents

This chapter provides tips, tricks, information on materials and manufacturing steps. These should be considered as suggestions.

8.1 Materials for the Production of Thermoplastic Splints

8.1.1 Thermoplastic Splint Materials

Thermoplastic materials, also known as low-temperature thermoplastics, are suitable for the production of splints that can be individually shaped and immediately adjusted. The material is heated at a water temperature of about 70°, reaching a soft, malleable state. Within 30–60 seconds, the material is molded to the hand and hardens during this process. The splint is then removed from the hand for further processing and completion. There is a wide range of different materials, which differ in stability, flexibility, processing and curing time.

We use the following for splint production:

8.1.1.1 Orfit® Colors NS

In addition to the diverse color selection, which is great for children, the material can be very well formed and stretched. Modeling of interdigital spaces and hand arches is easily possible. The material hardens in a very short time. The edges can be cut well. This material is available in thicknesses of 2.0 and 3.4 mm.

8.1.1.2 Orfit® Classic

Orfit® Classic exists in the thickness of 1.6 mm. It has a similar texture to Orfit® Colors NS and is suitable for the small hands of newborns, preemies or very delicate underdeveloped hands due to its low material thickness (Fig. 8.1a).

8.1.1.3 Ezeform™

Ezeform™ 3.2 mm. We tend to use this material when we need a high splint firmness (Fig. 8.1b). It has a medium stretchability. More strength is needed to shape the tough material. Since it has

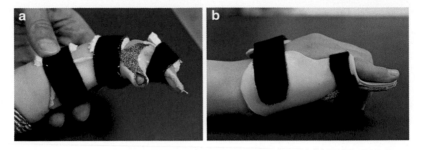

Fig. 8.1 **a** A forearm splint with enclosure of fingers 2–5 made of Orfit® Classic 1.6 mm material (white) and Orficast® (single layer/blue) for splinting the thumb. The materials can be connected. **b** A palm splint with enclosure of the little finger made of Ezeform™. Reinforcement with Orficast® (orange) gives the splint additional stability. (© Children's Hospital Wilhelmstift, with kind permission)

a high stiffness, this material is well suited for hands that have a strong contracture or a strong resistance, such as in children with camptodactyly (Chap. 4) and club hands (Chap. 2).

8.1.1.4 Orficast®

This material is self-adhesive after heating and has a high elasticity in two directions. It hardens quickly and due to its low material thickness, it is also suitable for infant hands as well as for individual fingers. To increase stability, the material can also be used in two or three layers. Orficast® can also be combined with other thermoplastic materials (Fig. 8.1a, b).

8.1.2   Fleece and Hook Tapes

8.1.2.1 Fleece Tapes

These are available in all possible colors and in different widths. They can be easily cut to the necessary size without losing their structure. Many fleece tapes have a firm texture on the outside and are fluffy on the inside (Fig. 8.2a, b). We use double-sided fleece tape for the production of infant or toddler splints or for reins between the fingers to prevent scratching injuries (Fig. 8.1a, b).

8.1.2.2 Self-Adhesive Velcro Tapes/Hook Tapes

Self-adhesive Velcro tapes/hook tapes can be individually cut and glued directly onto the thermoplastic splint. We always heat the adhesive side before attaching it to the splint with a hot air gun, this ensures better adhesion, which is especially useful for children.

If the Velcro tape is used for the Orficast®, a piece of Orficast® is glued to the adhesive side of the Velcro tape, heated and connected to the splint in the warm state.

8.1.3   Self-Adhesive Edge Pads

There are various self-adhesive pads. Depending on the deformity, the size of the child, and the area of the splint to be padded, the respective thickness is selected.

We use:

8.1.3.1 Eding Strip

For the encasement of splint edges. The edge strips **from Orfit®** are a thin (1 mm), stretchable, elastic, self-adhesive textile material.

8.1.3.2 Edge Pads from Cellona®

In 2 mm thickness. It is slightly stretchable in both directions and a self-adhesive padding material.

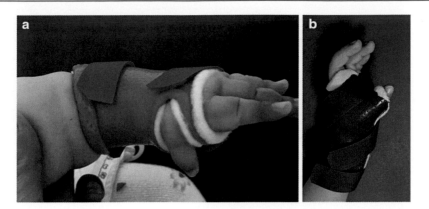

Fig. 8.2 **a** The white edge padding forms a buffer between the soft tissue and the splint, thus preventing pressure marks and edema. **b** The thin fleece fabric fits into the small structures of the pollicization splint and cushions the pressure points. This prevents pressure marks. (© Children's Hospital Wilhelmstift, with kind permission)

We use this for splint edges that enclose soft hypoplastic tissue such as in the case of a club-hand with thumb hypoplasia (Fig. 8.2a) (Chap. 2).

8.1.3.3   HAPLA Fleece Fabric from RUSSKA

It is a 1 mm thick self-adhesive fleece, stretch-able in one direction. It is made of 100% cotton and is hypoallergenic. We use this material, for example, to pad out a splint around a pollicized thumb and the first interdigital fold (Fig. 8.2b) (Chap. 3).

8.1.4   Padding as Spacers

We assemble a so-called spacer between the splint edges ourselves. A self-adhesive Velcro tape is glued onto a 4 mm thick cotton-coated pad, with the cotton side facing the child. This spacer is cut to fit the respective space between the splint edges and is attached to a fleece tape. When closing the fleece tape, the spacer is slightly pressed into the child's tissue between the splint edges. This prevents too tight a pull and the pressing of the edges into the child's tissue, and gives a limit to the tension strength when parents close the splint (Fig. 8.3a, b and 8.4).

8.1.5   Tubular Bandages

To obtain a thin layer of fabric between skin and splints, a tubular bandage of the respective width can be pulled under the splint. This prevents skin reactions due to, for example, sweat depos-its when renewed regularly. There are various manufacturers for this. To obtain thicker pad-ding, the tubular bandage can also be doubled (Fig. 8.4).

8.1.6   NRX Straps, Elastic Fleece Straps

NRX straps or elastic fleece straps have good stretchability in one direction. We use these, for example, for exercise splints to improve finger flexion, thus individual fingers are held in flex-ion with tension for up to 30 minutes.

8.1.7   Finger Loops/Fixation Bandages

We use finger loops and fixation bandages:

- to solidarize fingers,
- to restrain or fix fingers in the splint,
- to connect splint areas.

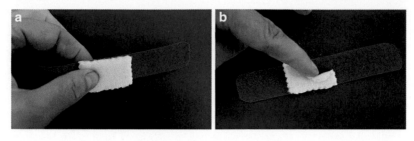

Fig. 8.3 a, b The spacer consists of a 4 mm thick coated pad, a self-adhesive Velcro tape was glued to the back and connected to the fleece tape. (© Children's Hospital Wilhelmstift, with kind permission)

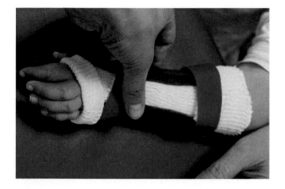

Fig. 8.4   Between the splint edges, under the blue fleece tapes, is the white spacer. To obtain padding between skin and splint and to avoid direct skin contact with the splint, the child wears a once-folded tubular bandage. (© Children's Hospital Wilhelmstift, with kind permission)

- Camptodactylies to restrain the little finger to the ring finger, to counteract ulnar deviation (Chap. 4) (Fig. 8.5a).
- Glove-Splints for the treatment of middle and ring fingers. The rein serves as a connection of the splint parts (Chap. 4) (Fig. 4.14 c, d).
- the aftercare following pollicization to restrain fingers 3–5 to prevent the interdigital grip or to force an opposition movement (Chap. 3) (Fig. 3.18 a, b) (Fig. 8.5b).
- the fixation of a finger in a splint. In this case, the outside of the loop is turned towards the child (as this side is velcro) and connected with the hook band (Chap. 3) (Fig. 4.20 d) (Fig. 8.5c).

8.1.7.2 Peha-haft®

Peha-haft® is an elastic fixation bandage, with a double adhesive effect. We use this material in aftercare to fix splints to malformed hands, for example. Due to the malformation, some hands have a conical anatomy, which means that the

8.1.7.1 Buddy Loop®

Buddy Loop® is a finger loop made of an inner foam and an outer velcro band. Due to its soft and elastic nature, we use the Buddy Loop® for:

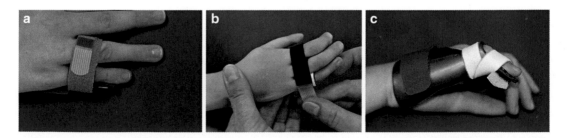

Fig. 8.5   a A rein that connects the little finger with the ring finger counteracts the ulnar deviation of the little finger. **b** Fingers 3–5 are fixed with a Buddy Loop® to prevent the interdigital grip. **c** A Buddy Loop® fixes the finger at the base of the finger and at the fingertip in the splint. (© Children's Hospital Wilhelmstift, with kind permission)

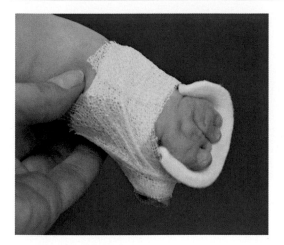

Fig. 8.6 To fix the splint to the conical hand, the forearm is first wrapped with Peha-haft® and after applying the splint, Peha-haft® is again wrapped over the splint. Both adhesive layers connect with each other and thus prevent the splint from slipping. (© Children's Hospital Wilhelmstift, with kind permission)

hand tapers off and without hardly any structure for fixing the splint.

First, Peha-haft® is wrapped around the arm and/or hand before the splint is applied, then the splint is applied and again fixed with Peha-haft®. Both Peha-haft® layers connect with each other and thus prevent slipping (Fig. 8.6). Peha-haft® can also be used to solidarise fingers. In this case, a piece of Peha-haft® is folded lengthwise and wrapped around the base joints to be fixed, it is recommended to start the wrapping between the fingers to prevent skin-to-skin contact. Peha-haft® can also be used to prevent the child from removing the splint independently. For this, the fleece bands are removed and the Peha-haft® is wrapped around the splint. The hook band serves for better anchoring of the bandage.

> **Cave:**
> The Peha-haft® must not be wrapped too tightly around the skin, as it tends to retract.

8.2   Materials and Manufacturing of Orthoses

Using an example:

Chapter 2/Fig. 2.16   a,   b/Preoperatively, 18-month-old boy, with RLD and left thumb hypoplasia.

Forearm orthosis with individual finger enclosure of fingers 2–5.

The hypoplastic thumb remains free, the flexion contractures of fingers 2–5 are corrected by the splint, and the wrist is straightened ulnarly and dorsally.

8.2.1   Plaster Cast (Negative Imprint)

8.2.1.1   Materials for Making a Plaster Cast

- Tape measure, possibly calipers
- Measurement sheet/pen
- Camera
- Lukewarm water/bowl
- Plaster
- Cream e.g. Vaseline for isolation
- Copy pencil
- Bandage scissors
- Silicone pad made of two-phase silicone*
- Sturdy plastic tube* or similar

Pre-made **silicone pads made of two-phase silicone** or two-component silicone can be used to make a plaster cast for a forearm-finger orthosis. Especially in infants and toddlers, the pad facilitates plastering, as the little ones usually do not keep still and automatically clench their fingers. The material is stable and slightly elastic and can be cut to shape (Fig. 8.7a). Silicone pads can be prepared on existing plaster models and the respective size for the patient can be selected (Fig. 8.7b). If fingers have significantly different contractures, individually adapted finger silicone pads facilitate the production of a good plaster imprint.

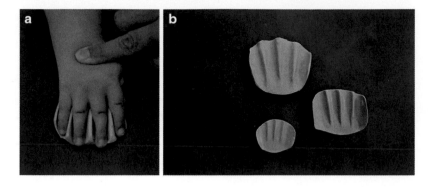

Fig. 8.7 a Pre-made finger pad made of 2-phase silicone, the fingers are placed at a sufficient distance from each other. **b** Pre-made finger pad, made on existing plaster models. (© Children's Hospital Wilhelmstift, with kind permission)

A **sturdy plastic tube** with a diameter of approx. 0.5 cm (e.g. from the aquarium shop), which is placed on the arm before plastering and removed after the plaster has hardened, forms a cutting channel for the bandage scissors (Fig. 8.8).

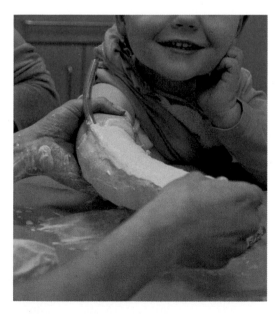

Fig. 8.8 After moisturizing the skin, the greased tube is placed on the skin. The soaked plaster bandages are wrapped around the arm and the tube. Once the plaster is firm enough, the tube is pulled out of the plaster, the resulting channel facilitates cutting. (© Children's Hospital Wilhelmstift, with kind permission)

8.2.1.2 Plaster Cast for the Creation of Orthoses with Individual Finger Enclosure

Preliminary Information

- The hand and fingers are photographed from the palmar, dorsal, and medial sides, in the spontaneous position and in the desired extension. Contracted fingers are photographed individually, the elbow with the forearm in a bent and extended position. This is followed by the measurement of the hand and forearm.
- The wrist and fingers are measured and documented in passive extension.

All this information serves as a control during the creation of the plaster model.

- The colors for the splints are chosen by the patients or parents.

Plastering

Before plastering, a pre-made finger guide made of 2-phase silicone is selected (Fig. 8.7a, b). This guide keeps the fingers at a sufficient distance from each other, prevents their bending, and facilitates holding during plastering. If the fingers are in significantly different flexion contractures, an individually adapted imprint made of 2-phase silicone is recommended. This imprint ensures a more precise working method when creating the plaster model.

Prominent areas and the base joints are marked with a copying pencil. These markings are later visible in the plaster model and help in assessing the finger position and serve as reference points when modeling. Now both the forearm and the hand are moisturized to make it easier to remove the plaster. An existing thumb is left out in the plaster imprint, but must definitely be moisturized. A greased tube, which serves as a cutting aid, is placed on the dorsal side and is fixed by the holder. With one hand, the elbow and the proximal forearm are enclosed and with the other, fingers 2–5 are enclosed in the existing finger pad while the hand is pulled distally and ulnarly and oriented dorsally.

With this holding function, both evasive movements by the child are prevented and the wrist is straightened.

The wet plaster bandage is rolled around the arm and hand without tension. Once these are circumferentially covered in a single layer, a four-layer plaster longuette is molded from the palmar side. Then another wet plaster bandage is wrapped around in a circular manner until the circular wrapping is four layers thick in total. Strong hand impressions, soft tissue displacements, and constrictions caused by the plaster bandage must be prevented. While the plaster hardens, the person making the plaster cast supports the holder by aligning the hand dorsally and modeling the hollow hand. Before opening the plaster, lines are drawn across the cutting aid with a copying pencil. This serves to close and maintain the shape of the plaster imprint after it has been removed. After removing the tube, the plaster is cut open through the resulting channel with bandage scissors. As soon as the child's hand has been removed from the plaster, the imprint is put back together and circularly wrapped with a thin layer of plaster.

8.2.2   Scanning for the Creation of Orthoses with Individual Finger Enclosure

Depending on the malformation and age of the child, the arm can be scanned instead of plastering. The patient must remain still during this process. Small adhesive dots are placed on prominent areas (e.g., ulnar head), fixed points, and pivot points, which serve as reference points for the technician during processing and highlight certain structures. Then, a series of photos are taken around the extremity using a 3D scanner, creating a three-dimensional image. On the PC, the 3D model is individually adjusted and the orthosis is constructed. A 3D printer prints the splint after processing. Various materials and printing methods are used, which vary depending on the desired properties of the orthosis.

8.2.3   Creation of the Plaster Model (Positive Print)

Before the plaster imprint is cast, the position of the silicone pad is checked. It remains in the plaster for casting, as it significantly determines the shape and course of the fingers. The plaster is now wrapped around in a circular manner, e.g., with a linen adhesive tape. A four-layer plaster longuette closes the cut. Here too, the position of the lines on the plaster impression should be taken into account to avoid an unwanted change in position. The plaster imprint is cast with a mixture of porous plaster and hard plaster. Before modeling, anatomical peculiarities and orientation points should be marked with small nails, e.g., the base joints and the ulnar head. The plaster is alternately removed and applied until it has reached the desired functional shape. The documented measurements and photos serve as a control and guideline. If the wrist position needs to be corrected further, this is done via the forearm and not via the hand to avoid affecting the finger position. For the individual finger guides or the webs, approx. 4 mm deep grooves are cut into the plaster model. They serve as spatial orientation during later welding of the webs. Before drying, the plaster surface is smoothed.

8.2.4 Manufacture of an Orthosis

8.2.4.1 Materials Needed to Create an Orthosis

- Streify-Flex©*
- Carbon*
- Orthosis finger pad (consisting of neoprene and Alveolux XRE©)*
- Deflection pulleys*

Streify-Flex© is a silicone-like plastic used for orthoses. The heated material is pulled over the plaster model. The seam must run dorsally over the back of the hand and forearm. It is then recommended to apply some additional Streify-Flex© (2 mm) in the hand area from the palmar side as a filler (for the grooves incorporated into the plaster model between the fingers). The hot material is then drawn to the plaster model using vacuum and thus takes its shape. (Tip: For orthoses without a carbon component,

it is advisable to additionally weld a reinforcement (4 mm) onto the palmar side, which provides more stability in the wrist.) After cooling, the palmar filler and the weld seam are ground down. The surface is smoothed. It is easy to work with, modify and adjust its stability and fit as needed or to form it thermoplastically. It is easy to clean. Due to the possibility of adding or removing material, it is particularly suitable for treating varying degrees of finger flexion contractures (Fig. 8.10). Tabs can also be welded on and opened due to the elasticity, to place the hand in the splint and enclose it circularly (Fig. 8.9a, b). This is particularly suitable for small, soft infant hands to guide the soft tissues. The circular enclosure prevents edge pressure on the skin and generates the largest possible contact surface.

Carbon is a plastic reinforced with carbon fiber, consisting of stretched carbon fibers that are bound in their position by laminating resin. It has extreme firmness and rigidity while being very lightweight. Carbon shells can be used to stabilize the Streify-Flex© orthoses, in which case the hard carbon shell is cast over the Streify-Flex©. In addition to stabilization, the carbon shell serves as an attachment for the straps (Fig. 8.9b). A half-shell design is recommended.

The **orthosis finger pad** consists of single-layer neoprene 3 mm and double-layer Alveolux XRE© each 4 mm. The Alveolux XRE© can be individually processed, which offers the

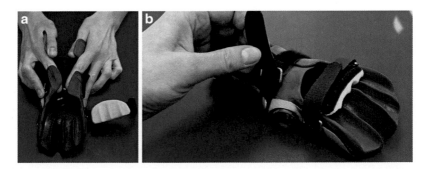

Fig. 8.9 a, b The splint is made of Streify-Flex©, the material is reinforced on the palmar side, the tabs run thin on the dorsal side. Due to the elasticity, the tabs can be fully opened. When closing, one tab lies under the other, which allows a circular closure of the splint. A half-shell carbon shell stabilizes the splint and serves as a holder for the straps. (© Children's Hospital Wilhelmstift, with kind permission)

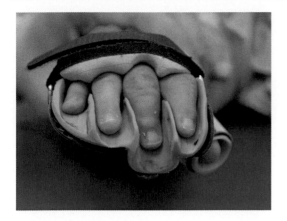

Fig. 8.10 The finger pad, consisting of neoprene (black) and Alveolux XRE© (beige), was worked out so that fingers 2-5 lie at the base joints in a 0° position. Due to the swollen middle joint of the middle finger, the Alveolux XRE© had to be generously ground away. (© Children's Hospital Wilhelmstift, with kind permission)

possibility to compensate for different finger circumferences, contractures etc. (Fig. 8.10). It is stable and at the same time elastic enough to guide the fingers and avoid pressure marks. It can be easily cleaned and disinfected.

The strap of the finger pad is guided over two **deflection pulleys** (ulnar and radial side). This ensures a centered pressure from the dorsal side and prevents a one-sided pull that could draw the fingers into a deviation (Fig. 8.11).

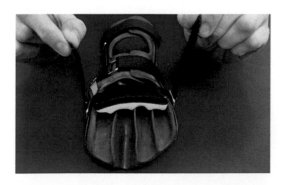

Fig. 8.11 The deflection pulleys for the finger pad are located on the ulnar and radial sides, since both tabs can be moved simultaneously, a centered pressure can be exerted on the fingers. (© Children's Hospital Wilhelmstift, with kind permission)

8.2.5   General Tips for the Orthosis

- The Streify-Flex material is thin on the dorsal side, which allows the tabs to be bent outwards, facilitating the insertion of the hand into the orthosis (Fig. 8.9a).
- The medial tab, which is placed under the lateral tab, must be smoothed over a long surface to avoid edge pressure (Fig. 8.9b).
- The finger bridges end proximal to the middle joints and taper from distal to proximal. They are high enough to support the fingers laterally but low enough to allow the pad to press the fingers into the orthosis.
- The orthosis can and should be cleaned every day with soap and rinsed with clear water, thus removing sweat and dirt deposits and preventing skin reactions.
- To avoid direct skin contact with the orthosis, tubular bandages can be worn under the orthosis.
- A forearm-hand cuff made of jersey fabric is made by our orthopedic technicians when the children have very soft tissue and, for example, the wrist is squeezed into extension by an orthosis joint. Due to the tissue displacement during stretching, the soft tissues can be bruised (Fig. 8.12a). This is prevented by the jersey fabric, which has slightly compressive properties (Fig. 8.12b, c). The plaster model is used as a reference for the cuff size.
- If wrist stretching is indicated in infancy or early childhood, a limitable Quengel joint for fingers often has to be used (Fig. 8.13), as all other orthosis joints are too large.
- If not only a forearm-palm orthosis is needed during the K-wire fixation after a radialization, but also a splinting of the fingers for nightly stretching, a forearm orthosis with removable finger attachment can be made. A knurled screw fixes the finger attachment to the forearm orthosis (Fig. 8.14a, b).

▶ The names Streify-Flex© and Alveolux XRE© are trademarks of Streifeneder ortho.production GmbH. The material Streify-Flex© originally comes from dentistry. The material

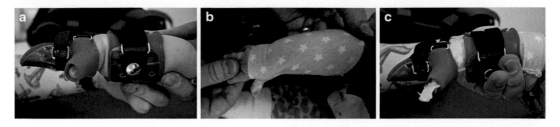

Fig. 8.12 a During the stretching of the wrist, the soft tissues are compressed and bruised on the dorsal side **b** An individually made cuff is pulled over the palm, thumb and the entire forearm. **c** The cuff compresses the tissue evenly. This reduces the compression of the dorsal soft tissues at the wrist area not covered by the splint during the stretching. (© Children's Hospital Wilhelmstift, with kind permission)

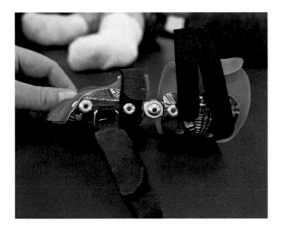

Fig. 8.13 A limitable Quengel joint for fingers serves as a wrist Quengel joint in infancy. (© Children's Hospital Wilhelmstift, with kind permission)

is LDPE (low-density polyethylene). The material Alveolux XRE© was developed by Streifeneder for orthopedic technology. For more information, please refer to the Streifeneder product catalog.

8.3 Dynamic Finger Extension/ Flexion Orthoses

We use the dynamic finger extension/flexion orthoses from Ruck MedicalTec© for stretching the proximal interphalangeal joint into flexion (Fig. 8.15a, b) or extension (Chap. 2 and 4). It serves as an exercise splint for short time intervals of 10–30 min (not longer, as the circulation is impaired by the strong squeezing). Through a small spring joint located at the level of the middle joint, the joint is stretched into the desired position and kept under tension (Fig. 8.15b and 8.5a). The half-shell guides, which encompass the base and middle phalanges, prevent rotational movements in the middle joint during stretching. To counteract a possible deviation in the base joint, the finger to be treated can be braced with a finger lying parallel (this can be done, for example, with a Buddy loop®) (Fig. 8.5a). If the finger to be treated turns a little redder than the other fingers after a

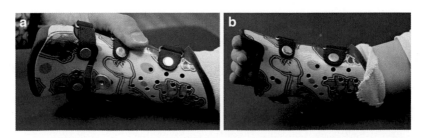

Fig. 8.14 a, b Forearm orthosis with removable finger attachment. During the day, the finger attachment is removed to allow for finger movements. (© Children's Hospital Wilhelmstift, with kind permission)

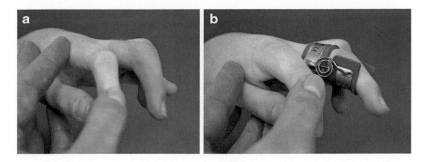

Fig. 8.15 **a** 13-year-old with pronounced flexion contractures of the proximal interphalangeal joints 3 and 4. **b** Treatment with a dynamic finger extension orthosis from Ruck, the orthosis is worn alternately on the fingers. (© Children's Hospital Wilhelmstift, with kind permission)

few seconds, the spring pressure is good. If the finger turns blue or white, the pressure must be reduced immediately. The pull of the spring can be increased or reduced using pliers. The circulation must be checked repeatedly during the time, especially in smaller children. If possible, the orthosis should be worn several times a day.

8.4   Definitions

8.4.1   Raising

When an orthosis is made to stretch or bend a joint, the orthosis material must be **raised** around the joint. This means that the material is modeled away from the child. Raising is also

necessary for static splints, especially when the children are very small, have soft tissue, and/or are very "chubby". This raised material serves as a guide for the soft tissues and prevents the formation of pressure marks (Fig. 8.16a, b). If the material were simply shortened instead of raised, the pressure mark would shift. Even with thermoplastic splints, edges are raised to guide the tissue or shift the pressure point, as is done with the splint for the Glove-Splint (Fig. 8.16c).

8.4.2   "Nose"

To expand the contact area for the hand during the day, a so-called **"nose"** can be made on the

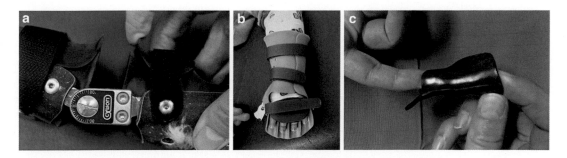

Fig. 8.16 **a** The Streify-Flex is raised around the wrist to guide the soft tissues that are pushed together during the stretching into extension. **b** For small "chubby" children, the material must be generously raised, especially at the proximal orthosis end, so that the soft tissues are guided and not pinched during the bending and extension of the elbow. **c** The thermoplastic finger splint is modeled/"raised" on the dorsal side at the level of the middle joint so that there is no pressure on the middle joint. (© Children's Hospital Wilhelmstift, with kind permission)

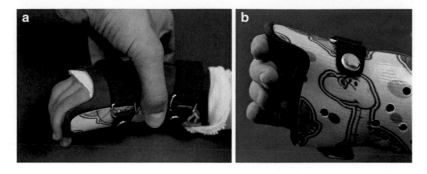

Fig. 8.17 **a** The "nose" on the orthosis expands the pressure contact area on the radial side. **b** The fingers are not restricted in their mobility by the "nose". (© Children's Hospital Wilhelmstift, with kind permission)

radial side of the splint. This "nose" increases the pressure contact area and thus the pressure distribution without restricting the movements of the fingers (Fig. 8.17a, b). This is particularly useful in the case of the malformation of the radial longitudinal reduction defect (Chap. 2), as the hand has a strong pull towards the radial side both pre- and postoperatively.

8.4.3   Extension System

The so-called **extension system** is used for pre-operative stretching of club hands (Fig. 8.19a–c) (Chap. 2). One pressure point of the three-point system is replaced by a constant pull (Fig. 8.18a, b). The upper arm and the elbow are fixed, and the hand is pulled distally and ulnarly with a lot

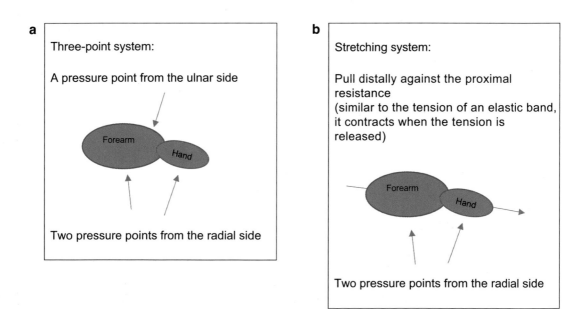

Fig. 8.18 **a** Three-point system. **b** Extension system. (© Children's Hospital Wilhelmstift, with kind permission)

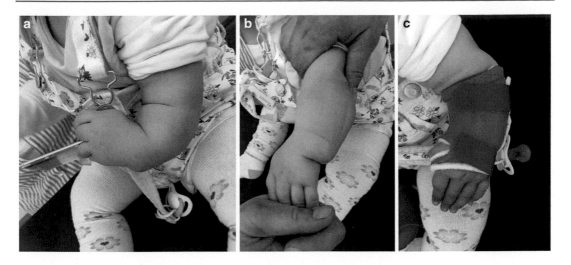

Fig. 8.19 **a** Club hand: Arm without stretching **b** Arm with maximum stretching **c** Arm in the brace shape, the extension system is established (© Children's Hospital Wilhelmstift, with kind permission)

of force and oriented dorsally. While the pull is maintained, a brace is modeled around the arm and hand from the radial side. The ulnar side is left out of the splint. As soon as the pre-stressed arm is released, it fits into the splint on the radial side, the "extension system" is established. The longitudinal pull is maintained in the splint, which has a brace shape (Fig. 8.19c).

Printed in the United States
by Baker & Taylor Publisher Services